HD
7264
.B37
1987

Barth, Peter S.,
1937

The tragedy of
black lung

$20.95

DATE			

The TRACEDY of BLACK LUNG

fEdERAL COMPENSATION foR occupATioNAL disEASE

Peter S. Barth

1987

W. E. Upjohn Institute for Employment Research

Library of Congress Cataloging-in-Publication Data

Barth, Peter S., 1937–
  The tragedy of black lung.

  1. Lungs—Dust diseases—Government policy—
United States. 2. Lungs—Dust diseases—Law and
legislation—United States. 3. Workers'
compensation—United States. I. Title.
HD7264.B37 1987   368.4'1   87-8332
ISBN 0-88099-045-7
ISBN 0-88099-044-9 (pbk.)

Dedication

This book is dedicated to my wife, Nancy J. Barth, who has consistently provided me with the support I needed to carry out this work.

The Author

Peter S. Barth is Professor of Economics and former Head of the Department of Economics, University of Connecticut. He is a graduate of Columbia College and holds a Ph.D. in economics from the University of Michigan. He was the Executive Director of the National Commission on State Workmen's Compensation Laws. He has been a Brookings Institution Economic Policy Fellow and a German Marshall Fund Fellow.

Aside from numerous articles he has written on workers' compensation, he has prepared special studies on asbestos compensation in Ontario, occupational disease compensation in New York, the use of impartial medical opinion in California cases, the experience of survivors of workers deceased due to asbestos-caused diseases, and the administration of workers' compensation in Connecticut. In 1980, he completed a study for the U.S. Department of Labor on medical panels in workers' compensation cases in Canada. A 1985 monograph on the use of medical panels was published by the Workers Compensation Research Institute. His book, *Workers' Compensation and Work-Related Illnesses and Diseases,* (MIT Press, 1980) was awarded the Kulp Memorial Prize for 1981 by the American Risk and Insurance Association.

Acknowledgments

Many people assisted in preparing this study, either by sharing their time or available materials with me. These include James Brown, James DeMarce, Robert Dorsey, Donald Elisburg, Judith Greenwood, Dr. Lorin Kerr, Lawrence Kovitch, Hervey Levin, Daniel Price, Donald Ridzon, Sydnee Schwartz and Mark Solomons.

Special thanks to the W. E. Upjohn Institute for Employment Research which was totally supportive at every step of the way, despite my frequently missed deadlines. The late Earl Wright encouraged me at the outset and H. Allan Hunt helped me finish up. Allan's comments on my early drafts were especially helpful. Judy Gentry of the Institute provided me with editorial support. Kristine Krause was a world class typist for me. I am solely responsible for any errors of omission or commission that follow.

Preface

Section 27 of the Occupational Safety and Health Act of 1970 provided for the establishment of a presidential commission to evaluate state workers' compensation laws. In 1972, the National Commission on State Workmen's Compensation Laws issued its report, which found many shortcomings and inadequacies in the state programs. It called upon the states to improve their laws and the administration of these programs, but urged that federally set minimum standards be imposed if these reforms were not implemented by 1975. The threat of such federal intervention in an area that traditionally had been left to the states caused many states to upgrade their programs dramatically, especially in the area of benefits. However, efforts to set and impose federal standards, which began in 1973, never succeeded in the Congress.

By the late 1970s, federal interest in state workers' compensation programs had shifted to the problems of occupational diseases. This had been prompted by a number of studies that appeared to demonstrate some major difficulties in the way the states were handling the compensation of workers or the survivors of workers who might have contracted an occupational illness. Compounding this was the upheaval created in about 1981 over growing numbers of workers' compensation and product liability claims involving asbestos exposure. Once more, there was a serious inclination shown by some in the U.S. Congress to legislate in the area of occupational disease compensation.

A variety of difficult issues had to be confronted in the course of the debate over federal involvement. Should the federal government impose standards on the states or should the state systems simply be supplanted in this area? Should such legislation deal with all occupational diseases or only with those specified in a statute? Would compensation be provided solely for newly emerging cases, or would cases be accepted where death or disability had occurred before the enactment of the law? Who was to bear financial responsibility for such a compensation program? Who would administer such a program? Could a federal program coexist with the state workers' compensation systems without somehow undermining them? Was legislation understood to be the

vii

forerunner of an eventual usurpation of the state programs, many of which had existed for about 70 years?

In the course of legislative skirmishing, answers to such questions appear to emerge more from ideology than from analysis or experience. Perhaps it is convenient or comfortable for the parties engaged in such debates to resort to some conventional wisdom rather than to a hard look at evidence. Possibly, the inevitable exigencies of time and a lack of available evidence account for the casual or superficial manner in which such tough questions are analyzed. Or possibly, legislative initiatives are navigating in totally uncharted areas.

Current or future debates regarding federal workers' compensation legislation need not deal with those issues *de novo*. Instead, the parties can turn to the experience of the Coal Mine Health and Safety Act (CMHSA) of 1969, which created a compensation program for victims of a specific type of occupational disease. That program's existence allows us to evaluate at least one model of how a federal compensation scheme operates. The purpose of this study is to describe and evaluate that program.

This study focuses primarily on the period 1969-1981. The CMHSA or Black Lung program was substantially modified in 1982 and later, and it is premature to detail that more recent experience. Moreover, by 1982 the program had largely accomplished the goals its supporters had set for it. Although the amendments of 1981 are referred to when necessary throughout the text, they are treated in this study almost as an epilogue.

The first chapter of the study provides an explanation of how the federal government wandered into the area of occupational disease compensation in 1969. The next chapter gives an outline of the legislation and an explanation of why the statute was modified in 1972 and again in 1977. The medical issues of black lung compensation are described in chapter 3. This leads to a discussion in chapter 4 of the standards of proof imposed in the law and by the agencies that administer the law. Administrative matters and insurance issues are the focus of chapter 5. The purpose of chapter 6 is to give the reader some idea of the dimensions of the program, including an idea of the numbers of beneficiaries, the size of benefits available, and the costs of the program. The concluding chapter includes a description of the 1981 amendments. Also, it contains some material drawn from evaluations of the program undertaken by the General Accounting Office, using source data that could not be made available to me.

In assessing any governmental program, a critical initial step is to properly specify what the goals of the program were. Depending upon one's choice in this, however, the program can be considered to have been either highly successful or a crushing failure. I leave it to the readers to make their own assessment. My own views, which have changed often during the preparation of this study, are summarized in chapter 7.

Peter S. Barth
Storrs, Connecticut
March 1987

Contents

• 1 •
The Development
of the Black Lung Act

Until early in the twentieth century, an employer's liability for compensating an employee who was disabled as a result of a workplace injury was determined in a civil action.[1] Similarly, the survivor of an employee killed on the job was entitled to compensation from the employer only as a result of winning a law suit. In either case, it was the claimant's burden to prove that the employer had been negligent, thereby causing the disability or death of the worker. Demonstrating negligence was no simple matter, as employers could rely on several potent lines of defense. Delays of several years in reaching some final judgment were commonplace, legal expenses were perceived as substantial, and decisions often appeared to be capricious. Even as claimants began winning more judgments at the turn of the century, a few large awards were made to some claimants while others received nothing.

Considerable pressure for reform grew during the first decade of the twentieth century. Rather than seek to modify the system of tort law, proposals started to build on a relatively new approach to compensating injured workers and survivors that had recently spread across much of industrialized Europe. Known as workmen's compensation,[2] the system appeared to represent a significant improvement for workers—and possibly for employers as well—in Germany, England and some other western European nations.

1

Beginning with Wisconsin and New York State in 1911, the various states began to adopt their own workers' compensation laws, thereby replacing the existing tort approach.

As each state enacted such a law, considerable variation appeared in terms of the administration of the system, coverage, benefits, insurance arrangements and so on. All the laws seemed to conform, more or less, to certain underlying principles, however. First, each system operated on a no-fault basis so that claimants no longer needed to prove employer negligence. Benefits were to be paid for disability or death "arising out of and in the course of employment," a phrase found in all of the state laws and closely mimicking language in the various European states. The no-fault feature of the laws led to the hope that compensation would be paid swiftly and with little or no controversy and litigation. Benefits were to be paid in proportion to the wages earned by the employee prior to disability or death. As a kind of *quid pro quo,* each of the state laws made workers' compensation the "exclusive remedy" of workers or survivors against their employers. Thus, employers became obligated to provide benefits under this new scheme, but they freed themselves of the threat of possible law suits by injured employees or their survivors.

As the states administered their workers' compensation laws, a number of difficulties emerged in the matter of claims for occupational diseases.[3] A common problem was the need to establish the cause of the disease that disabled or killed a worker. Another cause of dispute between claimants and defendants often involved the question of whether or not disease was even present. Contention could arise also over the identification of the disease itself, since the presence of one disease rather than another might be more likely to be found compensable by those administering the compensation system.

Until 1969, the compensation of workers or their survivors for industrial injuries or diseases had been left entirely to state governments in the United States.[4] Since the federal government played virtually no direct role in the employer-employee relationship at the time states began enacting these laws, there was no question that if workers' compensation laws were to be developed, they would be left in the hands of the states. Federal legislation in this area prior to the mid-1930s would almost certainly have been declared unconstitutional. As each state refined its own unique system of compensation, and as various interests arose that depended upon that system, any potential role for the federal government seemed to diminish. Yet despite its historic inactivity, in 1969 the federal government shifted from its historic position and passed legislation to provide compensation to a specific class of workers—coal miners—for a single specific occupational disease. The purpose of this chapter is to explain how that change occurred.

The Nature of the Coal Mining Industry

Several factors set coal mining apart from other industries as a source of employment. These differences are due to a variety of special circumstances surrounding this work. One of coal mining's special, though not unique, characteristics is the physical risk of harm associated with it. The industry has been widely regarded as dangerous. Best known perhaps are the large-scale disasters where scores of miners have died in a single accidental occurrence. Yet the nature of the work also contributes to smaller scale or individual incidents that lead to death or disability. For example, in the period 1926-30, the fatality rate in coal mining was almost 2 per million man-hours of work.[5] Assuming a 2,000 hour work year, about 1 worker in 250 would die in a mining accident each year. Though the rate had fallen to 0.84 fatalities per 1 million man-hours by 1969, the rate was still high—about 1 fatality annually for every 600 miners employed full time, or a rate 7-9 times greater than that for the entire employed workforce.[6] Recognition of the dangers was widespread.

A second characteristic of mining is its isolation, both geographically and culturally, from other areas of the nation. Coal is mined, generally, in remote regions that are rarely, if ever, seen by people from the more populated parts of the country. This implies that coal mining is more than simply an occupation. Instead, it represents a form of society that was not touched by developments in the balance of the nation for much of this century. Set apart in this way, miners have often been subject to different treatment and standards by government.

A third characteristic of mining is the secular decline that gripped the mining economy during the 1960s. Coal production that had been at 631 million tons in 1947 fell to below 500 million tons per year during the early 1960s and had not exceeded 560 million tons per year by 1969. Moreover, in the later years of this period, less coal was being taken from the more labor-intensive underground mines and, instead, was surface-mined. Surface mining was found primarily in the middle west and western states, meaning that mining in Appalachia was even more adversely affected. The price of domestic coal, measured in constant dollars, fell in most years from 1947 to 1969, and by 39 percent overall during this period.[7]

The changing sources of coal, along with its displacement by other forms of energy, had a tremendous impact on employment in the industry. Between 1950 and 1970, employment in coal mining declined by 70 percent, from 483,000 to 144,000.[8] In addition to the decline in the quantity of coal demanded and the relative shift to surface-mined coal, the sharp increase in labor productivity in below-ground mines contributed to the drop in employment (see table 1-1).

Table 1.1
Historical Trends in Bituminous Coal Mining

	Production (million tons)	Employment	Productivity (tons/workday)
1950	516.3	415,582	6.77
1951	533.7	372,897	7.04
1952	466.8	335,217	7.47
1953	457.3	293,106	8.17
1954	391.7	227,397	9.47
1955	464.6	225,093	9.84
1956	500.9	228,163	10.28
1957	492.7	228,635	10.59
1958	410.4	197,402	11.33
1959	412.0	179,636	12.22
1960	415.5	169,400	12.83
1961	403.0	150,474	13.87
1962	422.1	143,822	14.72
1963	458.9	141,646	15.83
1964	487.0	128,698	16.84
1965	512.1	133,732	17.52
1966	533.9	131,752	18.52
1967	552.6	131,523	19.17
1968	545.2	127,984	19.37
1969	560.5	124,532	19.90

SOURCE: The President's Commission on Coal, Staff Findings, March 1980, p. 47.

One of the results of all this change in the economics of coal mining was the severity of conditions for miners and their families. With little or no other employment alternatives in the coal mining areas, long-term unemployment and poverty were endemic there. The economic deterioration of the coal mine regions created a sense that a great injustice had been perpetrated against the miners. The difficulty that many of these workers had in being able to relocate into totally different types of employment resulted in very slow rates of mobility out of these depressed regions. Those persons who remained behind but had no work were those with the greatest handicaps in the labor market: limited skills, advanced age, or health problems.

The economic difficulties of both the individual miners and the regions created financial difficulties for unions also. Since the United Mine Workers' Welfare and Retirement Fund was largely financed by a royalty based on coal tonnage paid by the mine owners, revenues were inadequate to meet the growing demands placed upon them by increasing health care costs and increasing retirement rates. Consequently, the fund was forced to reduce or eliminate certain benefits during the 1950s and 1960s, including some that were formerly provided to disabled miners or to survivors of miners.[9]

The Federal Role in Coal Mine Health and Safety

It has been observed here already that one of the things that sets coal mining apart from other industries is its physical dangers. What role has government, at any level, played in attempting to reduce the risks of coal mine employment?

As early as 1865, a bill was introduced in Congress to create a Federal Mining Bureau. However, it was only after a series of disasters that the Bureau of Mines was created within the U.S. Department of the Interior in July of 1910.[10] The Bureau was charged with ". . .diligent investigation of the methods of mining, especially in relation to the safety of miners. . . ."[11] The act did not provide the Bureau any inspection authority. Indeed, the law explicitly denied all Bureau employees any right or authority in connection with the inspection or supervision of mines. Part of the Bureau's difficulty was remedied in Title I of the Federal Coal Mine Safety Act of 1941, which authorized the Bureau to make inspections and publicize its findings and recommendations. The Bureau was unable, however, to set safety standards, an area previously left to the states.

During a period of serious labor-management strife in 1946-47, the federal government operated a substantial portion of the country's coal mines. The government used its opportunity as an employer during this period to have Interior Secretary Krug reach an agreement with United Mine Workers president John L. Lewis on a federal Mine Safety Code. When the industry was returned to private ownership in 1947, the code became a guideline (but not a standard) for federal inspectors. Operators were free to comply or not. Mine operators and state mine agencies were asked (in 1947 in PL 328) by the federal government simply to report on the extent of compliance with the guidelines. Seventeen of the coal mining states cooperated fully in reporting, two others responded partially, and seven states did not cooperate to any extent.

In December 1951, an explosion in a coal mine in West Frankfort, Illinois, killed 119 miners. In the wake of the disaster, President Truman signed PL 552 in 1952, which made compliance with the Mine Safety Code mandatory in mines employing 15 workers or more. Federal inspectors were given the right to shut down dangerous mines. Subsequently, several efforts were made both to tighten up mine safety provisions and to eliminate the exclusion from coverage of the smaller mines (14 or fewer miners), including a bill that passed in the Senate but not in the House in 1960. It was only in 1966 that PL 89-376 accomplished these goals.

The shared responsibilities of federal and state inspectors created obvious administrative problems. The federal role was aimed at averting large-scale disasters. The states' safety responsibilities dealt more with practices and conditions that could involve injury or death to individual miners. Aside from federal-state differences, substantial interstate variations existed in inspection policies and standards.

Workers' Compensation for Coal Miners

For an industry with the great physical risks of coal mining, it is not surprising that workers' compensation has always been an important issue. With the enactment of the state laws, miners injured or killed in mine accidents had recourse to state workers' compensation programs in order to secure some indemnity and health care benefits. While benefits may have been short of generous, they were not different systematically from those available to workers in other industries.[12] However, the widely shared perception was that workers who were disabled or the survivors of those killed by dust diseases had little or no access to workers' compensation benefits.

The two states with sizable populations of miners that did provide compensation for coal mine dust diseases before 1969 were Pennsylvania and Alabama. In the former, benefits were provided under a distinct program for miners with pneumoconiosis and were lower and less favorable in several respects than benefits available under the regular workers' compensation law. A benefit ceiling of $75/month was set on the program. Under the special program enacted in Pennsylvania, about 25,000 miners received some compensation for coal workers' pneumoconiosis from January 1966 through early in 1969.[13] In Alabama, 1,318 cases of coal workers' pneumoconiosis were compensated between 1962 and 1966.[14] It was very difficult for coal miners to receive workers' compensation benefits for dust diseases in West Virginia, though some did for silicosis. Only in 1969 was the workers' compensation law there liberalized for dust diseases in coal workers.

In the late 1960s, little interest in workers' compensation programs had surfaced at a national level.[15] Concerns regarding state programs were not evident, especially in regard to the arcane matter of compensation for occupational disease. This was not the case, however, at the state level, particularly in West Viriginia, which was in a state of ferment. A grass roots movement that began to coalesce among the miners in 1968 had begun to move for (better) compensation for dust diseases suffered by coal miners. A series of resolutions was introduced at the United Mine Workers of America (UMWA) convention in 1968 by various local unions. They won endorsement easily from the convention. The issue had been given high visibility in West Virginia, particularly through the efforts of three physicians who worked closely with the miners there: Isadore Buff, a cardiologist; Donald Rasmussen of the Appalachian Regional Hospital in Beckley, West Virginia; and H. A. Wells.

Following the convention, negotiations occurred between the UMWA and the customary coalition of mine operators over a new labor-management contract. In early October 1968, the first nationwide strike in 16 years was called by the union, and an agreement followed on October 14, 1968. The new contract provided a number of improvements in wages and fringe benefits over the three years of the new contract, but it did not contain any new language regarding either safety or compensation for occupational disease. The 1968 contract was consistent in this respect with a long history of UMWA contracts that had concentrated on wages and fringe benefits of working miners, but showed little concern with issues of safety or occupational health. The "business as usual" practice by the union displayed some insensitivity to concerns regarding compensation and safety on the heels of the interest demonstrated by the membership at their convention less than five weeks prior to the signing of the new collective bargaining agreement. The issues of safety and health might have disappeared or been forgotten except that the Farmington disaster followed so closely on the heels of this new contract.

Concern about dust diseases and compensation for them was generated by the three West Virginia doctors and also by Ralph Nader. At the local level, interest was also stimulated and spread by young activists who had been drawn to Appalachia as VISTA workers (Volunteers in Service to America), or in a variety of Great Society antipoverty programs established primarily under the Office of Economic Opportunity. Believing that economic and social injustice had led first to disease and then to economic deprivation owing to the lack of compensation, these young persons provided both the energy and organizational skills that allowed local Black Lung Associations to be formed and to grow. The union was not considered an ally. Instead, it was perceived as a part of the same establishment that paid little or no attention to the plight of sick miners or their survivors. The black lung movement during 1968 must be understood to have been driven by a dynamic that was more than independent of the UMWA; in large measure it was hostile to the union and seen as a source of political threat to the union leadership.

The three physicians appeared in coal mining communities throughout West Virginia. Dr. Buff warned his audience that they all had black lung disease and that they would die from it.[16] Buff traveled with a pair of lungs that he showed to his audiences. Dr. Wells would participate in the same program, holding up dried, black tissue sections that he claimed were ". . .a slice of your brother's lungs."[17]

In January of 1969, a large rally was held by black lung advocates at the Charleston Civic Center to focus attention on the issue. In addition to the trio of physicians, Congressman Ken Hechler (D-W. Va.) spoke to the group and read a long letter sent by Ralph Nader. The targets for much of the rally were the mine operators, the medical establishment that did not acknowledge black lung as a disease, and the union, for its apparent lack of interest in issues of health and safety and compensation. The breach between much of the union's leadership and the miner activists of the black lung movement can be understood in terms of the political divisions that were operative in the UMWA at this time and the eventual challenge to the Tony Boyle presidency.[18]

Although black lung legislation had been proposed in the West Virginia legislature that session, by February 1969 no action had been taken. At this time a series of wildcat strikes in southern West Virginia had spread quickly through other mine fields in the state. The original causes of the strike are in dispute but the issue that prompted its widening was the demand by miners for black lung legislation. As the strike spread, miners traveled to Charleston to let state legislators know that they wanted an improved compensation law. Bringing enormous pressure on the governor and state legislators, the miners marched through the city, ringed the legislature, threatened continued shutdowns of the mines and eventually pushed through legislation that liberalized workers' compensation for coal miners with dust diseases. Only after Governor Arch Moore signed the legislation did most of the state's coal mines reopen in early March 1969.

The role played by the UMWA in the West Virginia black lung strike was a passive one at best, and actually was seen as less than supportive by the activists in the black lung movement. One reason given by the UMWA for its role was that it had sought federal rather than state legislation to deal with problems of safety, health and compensation. By being an inactive party in the black lung strike in West Virginia, the union unwittingly had allowed a dissident group to emerge that could challenge its leadership. Thus the UMWA was forced into a more active role in the development of federal legislation.

The Development of the Coal Mine Health and Safety Act of 1969

On November 20, 1968 an explosion occurred in a huge mine (subsequently described by some as the size of Manhattan Island) owned by the Consolidation Coal Company at Farmington, West Virginia. In a year that recorded 309 fatalities in the coal mines in 13 different states, 150 of which were in West Virginia alone, two things made Farmington different. First, the magnitude of the toll from a single accident exceeded anything that had occurred since the West Frankfort, Illinois disaster in 1961. Of the 99 miners under ground at the time of the explosion, 78 were entombed when the mine was sealed 10 days after the blast. Second, the prolonged process of search and rescue lent itself to massive media coverage. Farmington became subject to nightly reporting on the network news. Very extensive coverage was given to the story in *The New York Times* and other national press. Coal mine safety was not simply an issue for the coal mining states any longer. A strong sense developed, spurred by the attention given to this community, that something had to be done for the miners to assure their safety in the workplace.

There is little dispute that the Farmington disaster was the catalyst that moved Congress to act. A widely shared goal in the Congress was to enact improved coal mine safety legislation within a year of the date of the Farmington explosion. The political environment guaranteed that the public's revulsion regarding the death toll in the mines would have to be assuaged. Lyndon Johnson's administration had proposed stricter mine safety legislation prior to this disaster. Farmington assured that something would be done. The physical danger of coal mining combined with a sense of economic hardship, if not injustice, assured that some federal action would be forthcoming.

In speaking on the floor of the Senate, the feeling was well summarized by Senator Williams:

> The active miner of today who toils manfully deep in the bowels of the earth to produce about 15 tons of coal per day was, until recently, the forgotten man, but the tragedies of the past year and one-half have raised him high in the eye of the public. The people of this Nation have been shocked by these unfortunate events and have demanded, on his behalf, that government and industry do a great deal more—not just half-way measures—to improve his lot. The active miner of today is feeling the wonderful benefits that an aroused public can bestow on him. The bill before the Senate today (S.2917) is a tribute to this public awareness.[19]

The legislation that eventually emerged as the federal Coal Mine Health and Safety Act of 1969 (PL 91-173) was directed at improving the safety of coal mining by enlarging the role of the federal government in setting standards and inspections. The tragedy at Farmington was treated as the last straw that compelled the federal government to extend its jurisdiction into areas previously left to the states. Early versions of the legislation that was to work its way through the Congress made no mention of occupational disease, compensation or pensions for disabled miners or widows of miners. By all accounts, the portion of the law that dealt with these matters arose as an afterthought by some, in the process of drafting and redrafting the health and safety law.

Within three months of the Farmington disaster the Subcommittee on Labor of the Senate's Committee on Labor and Public Welfare opened hearings on coal mine health and safety legislation. Harrison Williams of New Jersey introduced a bill that embodied the views of the United Mine Workers. Senator Javits of New York proposed a bill that had support from the Nixon administration. Jennings Randolph of West Virginia also put forward a proposal. On July 31, 1969, a bill that earlier had been reported out of the subcommittee won approval of the Committee. The bill's focus was on prevention and contained no mention of compensation.

The obvious response by the Congress to Farmington was to legislate tighter safety standards and possibly deal with health issues as well. Any dissatisfaction with compensation, an area administered traditionally by a state government, was not a federal concern. Yet the success of the black lung movement in West Virginia would be harder to replicate in the other coal-producing states. The mood in Congress was one of seeking to demonstrate some sensitivity to the plight of the miners and their families. The UMWA leadership needed some legislative victories to validate its tactics to its own rank-and-file.

In September 1969, S 2917 was brought to the floor of the U.S. Senate by Senator Williams. It contained no reference to compensation. The first person to raise the issue publicly on the Senate floor was Senator Byrd (D-W. Virginia). Senator Williams responded that a "short-term program" could be handled "temporarily" by amending the bill directly on the Senate floor. The two senators agreed that a study of the matter could be conducted at the time that a temporary program might be put into place. Their exchange helps to convey the spirit of that time:

> Mr. Byrd of West Virginia: Mr. President, I would like to ask the able Senator from New Jersey a question as to what consideration, if any, was given to the possibility of having provisions included in the bill which would provide compensation for miners suffering from black lung who do not qualify for compensation under State law.
>
> The reason I ask the question is that I have been very interested in legislation which would provide for compensation to miners suffering from pulmonary diseases who are not covered by State statute. In West Virginia there are many miners suffering from black lung and other pulmonary diseases who do not qualify under State statutes for compensation.
>
> With this in mind, I gave considerable time to the development of proposed legislation which would provide Federal assistance in this area. I was able to work with Washington headquarters of the United Mineworkers of America in developing a proposed bill which would provide Federal assistance over a period of 20 years, with the Federal assistance decreasing, I believe, in the amount of 5 percent a year and the States picking up the additional costs annually, but with no cost to the coal industry. I have felt that if the Federal Government could provide assistance along this line, without additional cost to the industry, we would not incur the opposition of the industry, which is already heavily

burdened with overhead costs: but, at the same time, the Federal Government would be assuming some responsibility in this area, and I think it should assume such responsibility.

So it was with the advice and counsel and assistance of Mr. George Titler, vice president, and other officials of the United Mineworkers of America, that I was able to prepare the proposed legislation, and my senior colleagues, Senator Randolph, and I joined in co-sponsoring it.

As the able Senator from New Jersey will recall, I appeared before his subcommittee and testified in support of this measure. My first question, therefore, is, Was consideration given in the subcommittee deliberations to adding provisions dealing with compensation?

My second question is, What are the prospects for such legislation at this point being added by way of an amendment to this bill?

My third question is, If such prospects are not good, what encouragement or assurance could the able Senator give to the Senator from West Virginia as to the prospects for such legislation in the near future?

Mr. Williams of New Jersey: First, the committee did not have before it any proposed legislation dealing exclusively with workmen's compensation for black lung disease, pneumoconiosis. One of the bills, S. 1094, although it included provisions on this subject, had health and safety as its major thrust, I believe I am accurate when I state by recollection that the first time the attention of the committee was directly drawn to the need for compensation for men disabled by black lung disease was by the junior Senator from West Virginia (Mr. Byrd). Of course, it was my personal feeling as chairman of the subcommittee that this certainly should receive careful attention and, so far as the chairman was concerned, most sympathetic consideration.

As we continued our hearings and deliberations on the safety and health measure, we did not deal in any comprehensive way with this particular approach of compensation for the disease. As necessary as it is, it was not dealt with at that point to the extent that we were able to include it in the pending bill.

So far as amendments here are concerned, it would seem to me that it is now established that this disease, without preadventure, is associated with the dust in the coal mining process, that it is disabling, and that it should be a compensable disease.

I would believe that our committee responsibility should be to consider it in depth. In the meantime, if there were a way to deal with this temporarily through a measure to bring disability payments to men disabled by the disease, certainly I would try to find, even now, a way to deal with the emergency in a temporary fashion looking toward a comprehensive long-range program of compensation for men disabled by pneumoconiosis.

Mr. Byrd of West Virginia: Mr. President I thank the able Senator for his response. I understand his answer to be that it is quite possible that consideration might be given on the floor of the Senate to language which would establish a short-term program to assist coal miners who suffer from pulmonary diseases and who do not qualify under State statutes. Am I correct?

Mr. Williams of New Jersey: That is what I tried to convey to the Senator, yes.[20]

The following day, the two senators from W. Virginia met with the very powerful chairman of the House Committee on Education and Labor, Representative Carl Perkins of Kentucky. The senior Senator, Randolph, introduced amendments to S 2917, co-sponsored by Senator Byrd. One of these (Amendment #211), extended a federal workers' compensation law, the Longshoremen's and Harbor Workers' Compensation Act to coal miners not covered by a state workers' compensation law. The law was to become effective two years after the 31st day of December that followed the enactment of the law. It would provide compensation to miners who were disabled or died as a result of "respiratory disease," and whose state workers' compensation law did not "contain provisions substantially the same" as those contained in the Longshore Act. Benefits would be paid by the mine operators under insurance arrangements; however, where this was not done, the Secretary of Labor would make payments from an Employees' Benefit Fund (Sec. 714). The fund would be repaid by having the Secretary of Labor obtain the money from "the employer of the injured employee," but the amendment also provided for funding through general revenues (Sec. 714 (F) (4)).

This amendment also called for the Employees' Benefit Fund to pay benefits in cases where the miner or survivor had not received compensation previously, but would have been able to if the provisions in the amended Longshore Act had applied at the time. Thus, "old" cases were to be covered under this amendment, though compensation was to be paid only for the period of time after the effective date of the law.

Senators Randolph, Byrd, Javits, Williams and Yarborough co-sponsored Amendment #212, introduced at the same time as #211. It represented a significant compromise from 211 and in several ways showed the imprint of Senator Javits, one of whose goals was to keep temporary any federal benefits program for black lung. This amendment called for the states to administer a black lung program with funds provided from the federal trust fund established in the proposed law. The states would receive and adjudicate claims based on standards issued by the Secretary of Health, Education and Welfare. Benefits were to be paid to either of two types of claimants. First, benefits were to be paid to "any coal miner who is totally disabled and unable to be gainfully employed on the date of enactment of this Act due to complicated pneumoconiosis which arises out of, or in the course of, his employment in one or more of the Nation's coal mines." (Sec. 106) The second category of potential beneficiaries was "widows and children of any miner who, at the time of his death, was totally disabled and unable to be gainfully employed due to complicated pneumoconiosis arising out of, or in the course of, such employment." (Sec. 106)

Amendment 212 described the time horizon for this program as "a temporary and limited basis, interim emergency health disability benefits. . . ." (Sec. 106) Several elements stand out in this proposal. First, benefits were limited to old cases only, that is, where disability had already occurred prior to the enactment of the law. Benefits would cease to be paid by the federal Trust Fund by June 30, 1972 at the latest, with the states taking responsibility thereafter. The terms *temporary, limited* and *emergency* are sprinkled throughout the amendment. Death benefits were to be paid regardless of the cause of death, so long as the miner was totally disabled and unable to be gainfully employed at the time of death and was suffering from complicated pneumoconiosis. Similarly, benefits for living miners also were limited to the relatively few persons who were unable to work and were totally disabled due to complicated pneumoconiosis. Of note also is the terminology used, "arising out of or in the course of employment," a phrase that appears in every state's workers' compensation law. (In virtually every state, however, the word *and* appears in place of the word *or*.) This clearly tagged the law as a piece of workers' compensation legislation.

After a series of further amendments, compromises and a resolution of the major issue that delayed matters in the Senate, i.e., its authority to legislate a revenue-raising measure not initiated by the House of Representatives, the Senate passed a black lung amendment on September 30, 1969. The vote was 91-0 in favor of the amendment, which carried Senator Randolph's name, with nine senators not voting. This Senate version was Title V, Interim Emergency Coal Mine Health Disability Benefits, and was incorporated in the act that passed the Senate unanimously on October 2, 1969.

On September 23, Congressmen Dent, Perkins, Burton and 22 others introduced HR 13950, their proposed version of the Coal Mine Health and Safety Act. It followed months of work and debate within the House Labor Subcommittee. By October 3, 1969, the bill emerged from the House Committee on Education and Labor without amendment and had 83 sponsors. Section 112 of this bill dealt with compensation for death or total disability due to complicated pneumoconiosis.

Basically, it provided that general revenues would be provided by the U.S. Treasury to fund either grants to states or direct payments to beneficiaries by the Secretary of Labor where no agreement was made with a state. Payments were to be for retroactive cases and not for prospective ones. The compensation provision passed in committee by a vote of 25 to 9. In reporting on the bill, the committee made a point of describing section 112 as follows:

> This program of payment . . . is not a workmen's compensation plan. It is not intended to be so and it contains none of the characteristic features which mark any workmen's compensation plan. Moreover, it is clearly not intended to establish a federal prerogative or precedent in the area of payments for the death, injury or illness of workers. These provisions of the bill are a limited response in the form of emergency assistance to the miners who suffer from, and the widows of those who have died with, complicated pneumoconiosis.[21]

Yet, in justifying the section the committee appeared to contradict itself:

> One of the compelling reasons the committee found it necessary to include this program was the failure of the States to assume compensation responsibilities for the miners covered by this program. State laws are generally remiss in providing compensation for individuals who suffer an occupational disease as it is, and only one state—Pennsylvania—provides retroactive benefits to individuals disabled by pneumoconiosis.[22]

The House version used the traditional workers' compensation phraseology, ". . .arising out of or in the course of employment." (Sec. 112 (G) (1)) In that sense, the section looked something like a compensation act.

The bill was explicitly limited to workers employed in underground mines. It contained a rebuttable presumption that if a worker with complicated pneumoconiosis is or was employed for 10 years or longer in a coal mine, then the disease arose out of or in the course of employment. Moreover, all persons with complicated pneumoconiosis were deemed to be totally disabled.

Ten members of the Committee dissented from the majority's position on the bill. (Actually 12 did, but 2 of these supported section 112.) Several reasons for their dissatisfaction with the compensation provision were given. The core of their argument, however, was that such legislation represented a threat to state workers' compensation laws by providing a federal program where none had existed before. "We believe that the long-standing and ever improving State system of workmen's compensation will be in serious danger of ultimate reduction to a mere subordinate appendage of a federalized system of workmen's compensation or even of complete elimination."[23]

In one dissent, a compensation administrator from Maine who had testified earlier on the bill for the association of state workers' compensation administrators, the International Association of Industrial Accident Boards and Commissions (IAIABC), was quoted as saying:

> The bills under consideration call for abandonment of our 55 year-old workmen's compensation system. (And,) The health, safety, and well-being of all workers, with few exceptions, is a matter of state concern. Workmen's compensation administration is a professional specialty demanding experience and dedication and an intimate knowledge of local problems. This proposed legislation would replace local control with a centralized administration impairing development in the various regions of this country.[24]

That opposition to black lung legislation arose over the mere creation of a new compensation program was not surprising. Workers' compensation programs in the states provided the livelihood for many persons in the legal and health professions, for segments of the insurance industry and for state administrators. A growing federal involvement posed a legitimate threat to these groups at a time when federal programs were rapidly expanding into a host of areas once left to the states. It is a testimonial to the strength of these interest groups that so much of the opposition to the Coal Mine Health and Safety Act was directed at this one small piece of the proposed law, and that it was directed at the principle of compensation much more than at the details of it. As stated on the floor of the House by Congressman Scherle of Iowa in seeking to rid the bill of Section 112, the compensation provision, "If this section is not struck, it will be the first step toward the ultimate federalization of all workmen's compensation."[25]

One of the specifics in the law that did occupy lawmakers was the bill's funding. Several issues were critical for them. The difficulties of the coal industry in the years preceding 1969 were certainly well known to senators and congressmen from coal mining areas. Consequently, they hoped to avoid putting much of the burden of financing the benefits section of the law on the industry, especially at a time where the health and safety aspects of the law were certain to drive up production costs and reduce productivity in mines. Since black lung was thought to be exclusively a problem of the underground mines, a tax levied on coal production would shift some of the cost burden onto the surface mines, thereby relieving some of the potential costs to the underground sector. It would mean also that less of a competitive edge would be given to the surface mines *vis-a-vis* the underground mines. However, many of the black lung supporters in the Congress from states such as Kentucky, Pennsylvania and West Virginia were eager to have benefits paid out of general revenues of the U.S. Treasury.

On October 29, 1969, HR 13950 was debated on the floor of the House. Congressman Scherle of Iowa sought to amend it by dropping the compensation provision, Section 112. After that failed by a voice vote, he moved to have the bill recommitted, however that effort failed also. This led immediately to a vote on the bill, which passed 389-4. In an editorial, *The New York Times* applauded the action of the House and then predicted, "The Conference Committee should have a relatively easy task of reconciling the two versions now that both chambers have made clear their refusal to be sidetracked by the once omnipotent industry lobbyists."[26] This proved to be one of many predictions made about the program that later proved to be completely wrong.

In November of 1969, conferees from the House and Senate met in order to reconcile the differences in the bills passed by each house. What emerged was S 2917, a version that looked significantly different from either of the versions that had earlier passed in both chambers. Indeed, the differences were great enough for John Erlenborn, the ranking Republican in the House Committee that fashioned the bill, to ask on a point of order for the Speaker of the House to rule that the conference report not be accepted. The grounds for such a decision would have been that the final version of the law amended matters that had not been in disagreement in the House and Senate versions. Erlenborn's point of order was overruled, thereby setting up the vote in the House on the conferees' version of the bill.

Erlenborn's position had been a difficult one. His work on the Coal Mine Health and Safety law had been substantial and had led to a number of compromises by the majority. In exchange for that, Erlenborn had supported the bill including the black lung compensation provisions (Section 112). However, from his perspective the bill which was returned from conference to the House of Representatives had been substantially undermined. According to him, the conference made at least seven changes in areas where the two versions previously passed were not in conflict and that changed the law substantially. Foremost among these, although both houses had provided only for the compensation of *complicated pneumoconiosis,* the conference stipulated that benefits were for the far broader coverage of "diseases of the lung caused by dust." Thus compensation could be paid, presumably, for a wide range of diseases including simple pneumoconiosis, a condition that was far more prevalent than complicated pneumoconiosis.

Another important change was to obligate the coal mine operator to pay disability benefits where there was either no appropriate coverage under the state's compensation law, or where the Secretary of Labor had not approved the provisions of the state's law. It also added an obligation on mine operators to be covered under an insurance arrangement for such claims.

The conferee's bill also required the Secretary of Labor to pay for compensation where the mine operator was not insured or if the mine operator was no longer in business. A mine operator would be liable to the U.S. Government in a civil action for recovery of these funds.

The anger expressed by Erlenborn toward the conference and its report as dictated by the majority Democrats emerges clearly in the record of the floor debate. Using terms like "underhanded," "travesty" and "behind scenes dealing," he and fellow Republicans, such as Steiger and Esch, who had previously supported the House black lung provisions in committee and in the House vote, demonstrated their sense of having been sandbagged by House Democrats such as Perkins, Dent and Burton. Unable to win on the point of order, Erlenborn moved to recommit the bill but lost by

258-83, essentially guaranteeing the acceptance of the conference version of the bill. All of the controversy was directed at the black lung compensation portion of the law.

As the debate about the integrity of the conference wound down, the remaining discussion focused on the cost of the bill. The Nixon administration had promised to provide its thinking on the legislation, but had never developed a coherent position on it. Only after the two chambers of the Congress had passed their bills did the administration begin to play an active role. Strong threats emerged that the president might veto the legislation, partly on the matter of cost. Well after the Conference Committee had begun its work, and only four days before its final report was issued, Secretary of Interior Hickel wrote to Senator Javits, providing him with estimates of the cost of the benefits provision of the law. Based on the disability criteria used to determine eligibility, the Interior Department estimated that black lung legislation would cost between $155 million and $384 million in the first full year of the program, and between $1.2 billion and $3.0 billion cumulatively for 20 years.[27] Hickel's estimates were ridiculed by Carl Perkins on the grounds that they were provided hopelessly late in the legislative process, and for being excessively high, presumably for political reasons. Further, Perkins asserted that ". . .this legislation transcends petty arguments over costs."[28]

Additional criticism of the administration's stance was expressed by Congressman Dent: "At one point a senator came before us (the Senate-House Conference Committee) and told us that the cost would be as much as $180 million. Gentlemen, if you took every miner in these United States and if you paid him $5,000 a year and bought his wife a chinchilla coat, you would not spend that much money. Finally, after a little bit of fact finding, he came down to $154 million and yesterday he came down to $124 million."[29] Dent estimated that compensation for living miners could not conceivably exceed $32.3 million.

Hickel's estimates were attacked by another of the legislation's primary movers, Congressman Phillip Burton. He charged that the last minute cost figures were ". . .politically motivated and White House dictated . . . an ignoble effort to deny any meaningful help to black lung widows and miners. . . ."[30]

The administration provided virtually no support for Erlenborn and others who were fearful that the compensation provision had been carried too far. Ultimately, the Nixon White House argued simply that workers' compensation was a matter to be left for the states. In the absence of any leadership from the White House, the final bill was a creature of the Democratic majority in both Houses. The conference report was easily accepted in the House by a vote of 333-12 on December 17, 1969.

On December 18, the Senate took up the Conference Committee's report. Unlike the House, there was no disagreement voiced by members of the Senate. Senator Javits explained how the compromises had been reached with the House members of the conference. All of the discussion was centered on the black lung provisions. Senator Williams indicated that he anticipated that 50,000 claimants would receive federal benefits under the law.[31] Javits asserted that Secretary Hickel's cost estimates were wrong and that he estimated the cost of the program would be between $80 and $100 million and "certainly no more than $120 million per year."[32] The conference report was approved in the Senate without a roll call vote. It was signed by President Nixon, despite his previous threat to veto it, on December 23 and became law on December 30, 1969.

The passage of Title IV of the Coal Mine Health and Safety Act was a tribute to the legislative prowess and doggedness of a few key members of Congress. None played a more significant role in shaping the final outcome than did Carl Perkins of Kentucky. While the legislation's most fervent supporters came from coal mining areas, there were at least three prominent exceptions, Congressman Phillip Burton of California, Senator Harrison Williams of New Jersey, and Senator Jacob Javits of New York did not represent such areas. Support for Title IV was helped by the very prominent positions in the Congress held by certain senators and congressmen from the coal mining areas. Senator Jennings Randolph, who sat on the Subcommittee on Labor along with Schweiker (R-Pennsylvania) and Taft (R-Ohio), had been chairman of the Senate Public Works Committee, earning for himself the sobriquet, the "Prince of Pork." The ranking Republican on the committee was John Sherman Cooper of Kentucky. Senator Byrd of West Virginia also served on the Appropriations Committee, and at that time had begun to climb the ladder of his party's hierarchy, serving as secretary of the Senate Democratic Conference.

In the House, the key Education and Labor Committee was headed by Perkins, who had served in the House since 1948. Congressman Daniel Flood, representing the anthracite districts in Pennsylvania, was chairman of the Appropriations Committee for the Labor Department and Health, Education and Welfare and was the speaker pro tempore. Congressman Hechler, a Columbia University Ph.D., was chairman of the Subcommittee on Advanced Research and Technology. John Dent of Pennsylvania held no special position of influence in the House, but his previous experience as an attorney, a former coal company executive, and a local union president (United Rubber Workers #1875) was helpful. Ultimately, there was little reason to expect much opposition to a bill that was pushed by such Congressional heavyweights and that appeared to be relatively cheap, if not innocuous.

Summary

The arguments introduced above are directed at showing the special place that mining occupied in the public perception. A combination of very high physical risk, growing dissatisfaction with state safety regulations, and economic deterioration in the industry meant that federal policy providing special treatment for the miners was not a surprising development by the end of the 1960s. In addition, this willingness to give the miners some assistance or support must also be viewed against the backdrop of Lyndon Johnson's Great Society.

Beginning in 1964 and extending through the balance of that decade, a very broad range of public programs of cash, health care and other services and in-kind assistance was provided to specific clusters within the country. Targeted at groups from the unborn to the aged, at veterans, ex-offenders, the handicapped, Indians, inner-city residents, the rural poor and myriad other populations, the prevalent view appeared to be that government support could right all of the past ills of the society. By the late 1960s, miners were simply one group that had not yet shared much of this federal largess. Apparent shortcomings in state workers' compensation programs that uniquely impacted coal miners provided a potential opportunity, fortuitously, for Congress to demonstrate its beneficence. The federal government had an established history of enacting coal mine safety legislation after major mining disasters. Hence, it was hardly surprising that there was a major bill passed in 1969, following the Farmington explosion. It proved to be a convenient vehicle for doing something that provided income to the coal miner community. The presumed need of the law arose from inadequacies that were evident in state administered programs, both in terms of workplace safety and health, and in workers' compensation programs for occupational diseases.

NOTES

1. For a general background on workers' compensation systems and their development, see *Compendium on Workers' Compensation,* prepared by C. Arthur Williams, Jr. and Peter S. Barth, National Commission on State Workmen's Compensation Laws, Washington, D.C., 1973.

2. By the late 1970s, workers' compensation had become the more widely used term.

3. The issues are described in Peter S. Barth with H. Allan Hunt, *Workers' Compensation and Work-Related Illnesses and Diseases* (Cambridge: MIT Press, 1980).

4. Two exceptions need to be noted, though they hardly undermine this statement: a compensation law for federal government employees and one for persons employed in longshore work.

5. Data from *Coal Data Book,* the Mine Safety and Health Administration, the President's Commission on Coal, February 1980, p. 139.

6. A rich set of data on injuries and fatalities in coal mining from 1870 to 1966 is reproduced in *Legislative History of the Federal Coal Mine Health and Safety Act of 1969,* Part 1, prepared for the Subcommittee on Labor, U.S. Senate, August 1975, pp. 535-578.

7. *Coal Data Book,* p. 99.

8. Ibid., p. 127.

9. A description of this and the response in the mining communities can be found in Barbara Ellen Smith, *Digging Our Own Graves: Coal Miners and the Struggle Over Black Lung Disease,* doctoral dissertation, Brandeis University, 1981, pp. 225-242.

10. See *Legislative History,* Part 1.

11. Ibid., p. 129.

12. For an overall assessment of the quality of workers' compensation programs in the late 1960s and beginning of the 1970s, see *The Report of the National Commission on State Workmen's Compensation Laws,* U.S. Government Printing Office, Washington, D.C., 1971.

13. The cost of the program was $32 million in (fiscal year) 1968.

14. *Legislative History,* Part 1, p. 523.

15. An exception, as in so many matters, was Senator Jacob Javits, R-NY, who was responsible for the insertion of section 27 in the Occupational Safety and Health Act (1970), thereby creating a national commission to evaluate the state programs.

16. See Smith, *Digging Our Own Graves,* pp. 324-325.

17. Ibid.

18. Ibid. These issues are described at length in Smith's dissertation.

19. *Legislative History,* Part 1, pp. 511-512.

20. Ibid., pp. 348-350.

21. Ibid., p. 1043.

22. Ibid.

23. Ibid., p. 1101.

24. Ibid.

25. Ibid., p. 1267.

26. October 31, 1969.

27. See *Legislative History,* pp. 1575-1577.

28. Ibid., p. 1550.

29. Ibid., p. 1560.

30. Ibid., p. 1575.

31. Ibid., p. 1598.

32. Ibid., p. 1631.

• 2 •
Black Lung Law and Its Changes
1969–1981

The purpose of this chapter is to briefly outline the major areas of black lung law as it evolved from 1969 through 1981. Here, the most significant characteristics of the law of 1969 and the amendments of 1972 and 1977 are described. In the chapters that follow this one, more attention can be given to specific issues and how they were developed under black lung law.

Title IV of the Coal Mine Health and Safety Act of 1969 is the section of that rather large statute dealing with compensation. It is called "Black Lung Benefits," with hearsay crediting this name to Congressman Phillip Burton, a California Democrat who actively supported the legislation and the subsequent efforts to liberalize it. The term hardly had been used before this time and apparently the name was inserted in humor into the statute.

The title consists of three parts, with Part A consisting simply of a statement of findings and declarations and six very brief, though not insignificant, definitions. The remainder, Parts B and C, bifurcate the law on the basis of the time when claims for benefits were filed. Part B, "Claims for Benefits Filed on or Before December 31, 1972," was to be administered by the Secretary of the Department of Health, Education and Welfare, which meant by the Social Security Administration (SSA). By contrast, Part C, "Claims for

Benefits after December 31, 1972," was to be placed under the management of the U.S. Department of Labor. Subsequently, the dates noted above were changed, but Part B and Part C have always referred to the separate programs operated respectively by SSA and the Labor Department.

The broad and stated goal of Title IV was to provide benefits to coal miners who were totally disabled due to pneumoconiosis and to dependent survivors of miners who died from that disease. There was little question raised about the desirability of compensating either those persons whose disease may have disabled them long before the 1969 law was enacted or the survivors of those whose death occurred at an earlier time. Indeed, the primary purpose of SSA's involvement was to administer a program for these old cases. Once this existing backlog was dealt with, the program would become a workers' compensation program for newly developing victims, administered more or less by the Labor Department. It was the hope of the bill's architects that Part C would find the states providing entitlements and administration under their own individual workers' compensation laws, with the Department's role reduced to one of certifying that the state was in compliance with the federal standards created in the 1969 statute. Thus, SSA's administrative responsibility for the program was a temporary one, to be turned over to the Labor Department, whose responsibilities were to diminish. Indeed, the latter's role was expected to be entirely eliminated eventually.

The Part B program provided cash benefits to miners totally disabled due to pneumoconiosis arising out of coal mine employment and to survivors of miners who had died from the disease. The program was funded by the general revenues of the U.S. Treasury (and not by the social security trust funds). To assist applicants in furthering their claims, certain presumptions, including an irrebuttable one, were included in the statute. Claims were filed in local social security offices.

Several of the characteristics of benefits under the law seem noteworthy. First, unlike workers' compensation or social security benefits (old age or disability), monthly benefits paid to successful claimants were invariant with respect to the miner's or survivor's age, the previous level of miner earnings, or the extent of impairment—although benefits were provided only for those judged to be totally disabled. Benefit levels were adjusted for the number of dependents, however. In most cases, benefits were awarded and paid for a lifetime. Benefits were awarded based on the date the claim was filed, not on the date when total disability began or death occurred. Since it was possible to be found totally disabled even though still actively employed in a mine or elsewhere, the social security earnings test was applied so that some or all of the cash benefits could be offset due to wage income. Offsets were applied as well to benefits miners received from state workers' compensation, unemployment insurance or temporary disability programs. Since SSA considered the benefits to be workers' compensation, benefits were also offset by receipt of social security disability insurance. Benefit levels were tied to federal employee salary scales, so that both new awards or continuing payments rose *pari passu* with federal pay levels and roughly, at least, with rates of inflation.

The Part B program was to accept claims for two years. The (virtually) lifetime benefits paid by the federal government under Part B were to be paid only for those successful claimants who filed no later than December 31, 1971, or where the miner died on or before that date, or finally, where a miner, who was entitled to Part B benefits, died leaving a survivor. Initially, 1972 was to be a year of transition. Successful claims filed during that year were to be paid by SSA only until the end of the year, with payment thereafter becoming the administrative responsibility of the Labor Department and possibly the states.

Essentially, liability for claims filed during this phasing-in period of 1972 were to be paid by coal mine operators beginning in 1973 under either Part C or federally certified state workers' programs, as were those claims filed after December 31, 1972. Presumably, the claims filed during the transition year of 1972 and later would reflect cases where the disease had only recently emerged. The hope was that all of the "old" cases would have been filed and dealt with in 1970 and 1971.

Some newly developing cases could be expected in the future, but by 1972 and beyond, the number was expected to be quite small, given the teeth in the dust suppression provisions of the new Coal Mine Health and Safety Act. Where new cases were not paid under acceptable state workers' compensation laws, they would be paid by individual mine operators. Where benefits from neither source were forthcoming, federal general revenues would be used. Aside from the continuing benefits paid to successful claimants under the Part B program, federal involvement in black lung compensation was to cease seven years after the law's enactment, that is, by December 30, 1976.

Since the 1969 law made individual coal mine operators liable for the benefits to be paid under the Part C program, the mine operators were required to obtain insurance to assure that successful claimants would be compensated. This obligation could be met either through a private insurance carrier authorized by the state to sell workers' compensation insurance, a state insurance fund, or through self-insurance where qualified by the Secretary of Labor. Where a worthy claimant was unable to receive benefits from a coal mine operator, e.g., the operator had ceased to exist and no insurance was available, benefits were to be paid by the Secretary of Labor out of general revenues of the U.S. Treasury. Unlike the (virtual) lifetime benefits provided under Part B, no benefits were required to be paid after the Part C program ended at the close of 1976. Thus, mine operators' liability was temporary—limited to four years (1973-1976)—although individual state workers' compensation laws were expected to fill in thereafter.

In order to assist claimants and to ease the burden of administering the law, three presumptions were inserted into the statute. Most significant was section 411 (c) (3), which created an irrebuttable presumption that evidence of *complicated* pneumoconiosis meant that either the living miner was totally disabled due to pneumoconiosis, or that the deceased miner's death was due to the disease.

The Social Security Administration was handed the responsibility for administering a law that was utterly new to it. For several reasons, including the specificity of the disease and the population covered, the Part B program bore almost no similarity to its disability insurance program. The 1969 statute left myriad issues to the discretion of the Secretary of Health, Education and Welfare, and a number of matters seemed never to have been considered by the Congress in its haste to legislate reform by the anniversary of the Farmington explosion. Of all the uncertainties associated with the new program, however, perhaps the greatest was the one regarding the dimensions of the program. However, SSA would not have long to wait before some idea of the size of the applicant pool materialized. Indeed, it was precisely this realization, along with one other development, that profoundly reshaped the character of the 1969 law.

Almost as soon as the law was enacted, claims began to flood into local social security offices. The same individuals and groups responsible for the passage of Title IV sought to encourage potential beneficiaries to file claims. These included representatives of the Black Lung Associations and the United Mine Workers of America, along with elected officials, antipoverty workers and to some extent, SSA itself. Undoubtedly, part of the effort by these groups was motivated by a concern to help the needy victims of the disease. Some of it was generated by those hoping to receive some of the credit for the existence of a law that would pump substantial sums of money into coal mining communities. Individuals who assisted miners or survivors in the filing of claims, primarily local attorneys and Black Lung Association representatives, had a financial stake in generating activity under the law. Finally, time was essential since benefits were paid from the date of the filing of the claims, and not the date of death or disability. Delays in filing would mean a direct decline in the value of one's benefits.

In the first year of the law, approximately one-quarter of a million claims were filed. By December 31, 1971, approximately 350,000 claims for black lung benefits were received by SSA. At the end of 1971—two years into the term of the law—new claims were being filed at the rate of 1,800 a week.

If the law of 1969 had remained unchanged, a massive potential liability would have awaited coal mine operators in 1973, based on claims filed in 1972 and thereafter. It also appeared evident by 1971 that the belief that the old cases would have been fully dealt with under Part B was unwarranted. As claims continued to pour in, the large bulk of them involved disability or death that occurred in earlier years.

It was not simply the massive number of claims, and especially the continued inflow of old cases, that concerned those members of Congress who were closely watching the development of the program. Senators and representatives who were strongly supportive of the law became increasingly dissatisfied with SSA's administration of it. To be sure, the agency had moved very swiftly to carry out the provisions of the law and render determinations. By the end of 1971, SSA had made determinations in almost 93 percent of the claims filed with it, despite the continuing flow of new claims being made. However, about half the claims made during these first two years had been rejected by SSA. Anger and resentment toward the agency by the coal mining community and their elected representatives over the rate of denials was substantial. In actively encouraging older miners and survivors to file claims, the law's supporters had given little consideration to the possibility that benefits would not be paid.

The consequences of the unforeseen volume of old cases, along with the disappointment over the rejection rate, caused the program's supporters to push for changes in the law. An obvious need existed, in any case, to amend the law to correct an error or oversight in the original act. Dependent surviving children of miners were able to receive benefits only where there existed a surviving spouse. Somehow, the language of the original law neglected to provide for "double orphans." There was no objection in the Congress to reopening the law to provide for these persons.

The prime mover in amending the law of 1969 was Representative Perkins. On the Senate side, Senators Williams, Javits and Randolph played a key role in reshaping the law. Ultimately, a reluctant Richard Nixon signed into law PL 92-303 in May 1972, following a unanimous vote in the Senate and an overwhelming vote in the House of Representatives (311-79). Its passage represented another clear-cut victory for supporters of the original legislation who hoped to liberalize its provisions further—largely, though not entirely, representatives from the coal mining states. Clearly, support came from more than Congressional liberals and/or Democrats. While supportive of the liberalization, a continuing concern of Senator Javits of New York was to place as much responsibility as possible on the mine operators. In his view, the entire problem reflected the ". . .accumulated injustice of not having adequate workmen's compensation laws on the books for years. . . ."[1] Perhaps his words were being directed to the National Commission on State Workmen's Compensation Laws, which was created through the Senator's efforts and was deliberating at that very time over the future of the state programs.

Republican Senators such as Taft (Ohio) and Schweiker (Pennsylvania) spoke enthusiastically for the bill that passed the Senate, as did influential Democrats including the Senators from West Virginia—Byrd and Randolph. The coal mine operators were behind the law, so long as it delayed the time when they would have to bear the financial responsibility for successful claims. The United Mine Workers were behind the bill solidly also. The recently elected president of the union, Arnold Miller, had received substantial support in his election drive from Black Lung Association groups.

The reconciliation by the Conference Committee of the Senate and House versions of the amendments was less dramatic or "creative" than it had been in 1969. Differences between the chambers tended to be resolved by selecting the more liberal provision or by splitting the difference between the two bills where that was feasible.

The amendments of 1972 were significant in several respects. The foremost of these was that the amendments served to clarify for all parties, and particularly for SSA, the agency administering the law, the intent of Congress. That is, the law's supporters wanted much more than simply to have *created* a new entitlements program. Rather, they wanted a program that actually delivered benefits to their constituents.

The huge and continuing inflow of claims, including many based on employment that ended prior to 1970, caused Congress to extend the dates of the act in several respects in the 1972 amendments. The House sought to extend Part B for two additional years so that it would run until December 31, 1974. This would have delayed the coal industry's financial liability accordingly. Further, the House sought to move the original seven-year federal role under sec. 422 (e) (3) to nine years, the period after which no benefits had to be provided under Part C. When the Senate voted to extend Part B for one year, the conferees split the difference and extended it for 18 months. The Senate voted to make the federal role under Part C a permanent one and the conference voted in a compromise to keep it until December 31, 1981. After that date, no payments to miners or their dependents were required under Part C of the law. Presumably, state laws would protect claimants who had filed for benefits only in 1972 or thereafter.

The conference also agreed that the transition period, originally planned to operate in 1972, would run from July 1, 1973 to December 31, 1973. As such, claims filed prior to July 1, 1973 involved lifetime benefits for miners or their widows paid by the federal government; claims filed after December 31, 1973 were the industry's full responsibility, and those filed in this six-month gap were to be temporarily a federal responsibility administered by DOL and then a private responsibility.

The 1972 amendments substantially widened coverage under the law by redefining both "miners" and "total disability." The revised statute added a new presumption which effectively expanded the meaning of pneumoconiosis. It enlarged the coverage of survivors, thereby widening the scope of the entitlements. It eliminated one of the financial offsets that had been applied to black lung benefits and made the change retroactive to 1969.

The 1972 amendments eased the burden of proof on claimants by preventing the government from denying a claim solely on the basis of X-ray evidence. In so doing, it effectively widened the range of impairments that could produce an entitlement under the law.

Possibly the most significant change of all occurred as a consequence of the amendment process, but it was not reflected in the revised statute itself. In brief, SSA agreed to revise the medical criteria it used to determine whether a claimant was totally disabled due to pneumoconiosis. Essentially, the agency promised to revise its published regulations in such ways as to assure that a larger proportion of claims would be accepted. Since the impact of these and all other changes were made retroactive, SSA was required to review all pending and previously denied claims using these new standards. This involved almost 195,000 claims, 90 percent of which had been rejected previously by the agency.

If the law's most ardent advocates were somewhat disappointed with its track record until 1972, they were devastated by developments after the enactment of the amendments. While SSA proved to be entirely accommodating to the liberalization of the law, on July 1, 1973 administrative responsibility for it shifted away from SSA to the Labor Department. The Part C program quickly became a disaster for the agency and the law's supporters. Over the next four years, six sets of problems became clear to all parties concerned with black lung legislation.

First, claims flowed in under section 415 (the six-month transition phase) and Part C in very large volume. Moreover, the bulk of these represented old cases, not recent or newly emerging diseases. The volume of cases had implications for both the future costs of the program as well as for the administration of those claims.

A second factor that became clear during this period was that the states were not replacing the Labor Department in the administration of the law. Few states applied to the Secretary to have their workers' compensation programs certified as acceptable to replace the federal scheme. No state ever received certification, so this vision of how the program would develop never materialized.

The third essential characteristic of the program that emerged under Part C was the litigiousness of those involved. The Part C program sought to place financial liability on specific coal mine operators. Also, unlike Part B, this was a workers' compensation program with an adversary process involved, and employers aggressively defended claims. In virtually every instance where a determination was made that an employer (or the insurer) should pay compensation, the matter was appealed.

A fourth characteristic of the program was that the Department of Labor, almost alone, was paying benefits under the program. In more than two out of three cases where benefits were awarded, no responsible mine operator could be identified or made liable. Moreover, where the appeals process meant that a mine operator would not pay benefits, these were paid by the Labor Department as well, though repayment was anticipated.

These four characteristics aside, there were two others that made matters particularly intolerable to the supporters of the program. One of these was the phenomenal delays that developed in the Labor Department in making determinations. Partly due to the unexpected outpouring of claims, partly due to the nature of the adversary process, and combined with the inexperience of and perhaps the ineptitude in the Labor Department, the system became totally backed up. From July 1, 1973 to December 31, 1977, no determination had been made in about 50,000 of the 123,000 cases filed.

The final straw, however, for the program's supporters was the approval rate in the Labor Department. By early 1978 (at the time that the 1977 amendments became effective), about 125,000 claims had been submitted to the Labor Department, with 6,000 awards made and 70,000 claims denied! Thus, in administering the law that the Congress handed it in 1973, the Department had been able to accept fewer than 8 percent of the claims received where a decision had been rendered, and most of these had had to be paid by the federal government rather than by the coal mine operators. To make matters even grimmer for the Labor Department, SSA had been able, by that time, to bring its approval rate under the Part B program up to 70 percent.

The Labor Department's track record was not a result of more restrictive policymakers there than in SSA. Rather, they were administering Part C with a different set of rules; the law gave them little choice, or at least so they believed. By 1975, Congressman Perkins and other black lung advocates worked to increase the number and proportion of applicants who would win awards. One means of pressuring the Labor Department was to hold hearings on the program and to continue to press for new amendments to further open up the law. Much of the work on the House side involved working closely with representatives of the Black Lung Associations, and the United Mine Workers. In 1975, Perkins pushed legislation that would have provided benefits for black lung based solely on 15 years employment in the mines.[2] Eventually, this was softened so that an automatic entitlement would occur for any coal miner after 30 years of employment in the mines. Such a version was actually voted upon favorably at one point by the House of Representatives.

In 1976, Representative Perkins and the Black Lung Associations pushed HR 10760, which created an automatic entitlement to benefits for miners with 30 years of work in the mines (or 25 years in the anthracite fields). Supporters of the bill argued that it was not a pension bill for miners, but instead that it reflected the very great propensity for long-term coal miners to develop black lung. Such a presumption would eliminate errors in claims adjudication and simplify processing them. The Senate was unable to act in a timely manner on HR 10760, but a similar bill, HR 4544 was introduced the following year. Largely with an eye on the Senate and on some public reaction to HR 10760, and realizing alternatives existed to accomplish this same goal, the House cleared a version of the bill on September 19, 1977 that dropped the controversial automatic entitlement. The Senate cleared its bill on the following day. The reconciled version that emerged from the Conference Committee sailed through both Houses and was signed by President Carter. In fact, to deal with the concerns about the implementation of Part C, two new laws emerged.

The Black Lung Benefits Reform Act of 1977, PL 95-239 (actually signed March 1, 1978) was a set of sweeping changes in the law. A primary goal of the law was to ease the burden on claimants seeking benefits for death or total disability due to pneumoconiosis. This was accomplished in several ways. Probably foremost among these, the Department of Labor was finally enabled to set its own medical standards, as well as to set temporary standards. Until permanent ones were developed, though, these temporary ones were explicitly to be no more restrictive than those set by SSA under the Part B program after the 1972 amendments. Recall that SSA had put in these post-1972 standards in order to raise the acceptance rate for Part B claims.

The law eased the problem for claimants of providing satisfactory evidence in several other ways. It eliminated the critical role played, until then, by specially certified experts, working as consultant radiologists for the Labor Department. Further, in the absence of other (medical) evidence, survivors could support claims by submitting affidavits regarding a deceased miner's condition prior to death. Autopsy reports by local physicians had to be accepted as evidence by the Secretary of Labor beginning in 1978. Some time limitations regarding the filing of claims were dropped. Certain restrictions on the use of the 15-year presumption that was added by the 1972 amendments were dropped, making the presumption usable by more claimants. Additionally, a rebuttable presumption that the miner was disabled due to pneumoconiosis was added for survivors claims where the worker was employed 25 years or more and died prior to June 30, 1971.

The concept of total disability was substantially broadened by several provisions of the law. For example, the Department was prohibited from using employment in the coal mines as evidence that the miner was not totally disabled at the time of death or of filing. The scope of coverage was further widened by adding three occupational categories and by significantly redefining the relevant workplace covered.

Prior to the 1977 amendments, the Part C program was to be terminated by December 30, 1981. This had been stretched out in 1972, so that the original termination date of 1976 had been pushed back five more years. In 1977, the provision that identified an ending date for the Part C program (section 422 (c) (3)) was eliminated, thereby appearing to make the program permanent. With improved dust conditions anticipated due to the Coal Mine Health and Safety Act of 1969 and its amendments, and with the states expected to be fully in line to replace the Part C program, the termination of the federal role had seemed reasonable at one time. Since the latter had clearly not occurred and since doubts existed about the potential for eliminating black lung disease, Congress chose to drop any pretense that this was only a temporary federal program.

To make its intent perfectly clear, the 1977 amendments required the Labor Department to re-review all claims previously denied and to evaluate them, along with the tens of thousands of pending cases, based on the new amendments. Moreover, new information could be provided by claimants who had been denied. Claims previously denied under Part B were to be reviewed again as well, though SSA's review needed only to have been based on the existing file. If a previously denied claimant, or one denied after the new review by SSA, wished to submit new material or evidence, that file would then be evaluated by the Labor Department.

The goal of the Black Lung Benefits Reform Act was to raise the probability that a miner or survivor would receive compensation under the program. But it did not deal with a central issue of liability, that is, the source of funding. Since the large majority of cases under Part C were ones where no "responsible operator" could be identified, and employers were vigorously contesting liability where they were so designated, almost all payments under the Department of Labor program came from the U.S. Treasury. Recall, that the original concept of the 1969 law had been that the Treasury would pay for the old cases only, and that the mine operators would be responsible for very recent and newly emerging ones beginning with claims made after 1971. Senators and congressmen from the mining areas particularly had been sensitive to the economically precarious position of the coal industry by 1969 and thereafter and did not want to burden it with substantial new costs for compensation. The 1972 amendments deferred the time when the mine operators would have to begin paying for black lung. And by

1977, very little payment had been made by them in any case. In defense of the industry, however, many of the Part C (and section 415) claims were based on employment in the mines that had occurred many years earlier.

To deal with the issue of liability, the Congress opted for a "superfund" approach, with the passage of the Black Lung Benefits Revenue Act of 1977, PL 95-227. Signed into law on February 10, 1978, the new statute levied a tonnage tax to be paid by all coal producers. These funds went to a federal Trust Fund to be used to pay benefits in three categories of claims. First, the Trust Fund was to be responsible where the Labor Department did not identify a "responsible operator." Second, the Trust Fund would be liable to pay successful claimants where the last employment in the mines had occurred prior to January 1, 1970. Thus, the coal mining industry now became financially responsible for the very old cases, though no single operator would be required to pay in these old cases. Finally, the Trust Fund would make payments where a benefit was awarded but the designated responsible operator did not pay in a timely manner. The Trust Fund would then seek repayment by the mine operator.

The creation of the new Trust Fund raised several intriguing questions. Was the tonnage tax rate to be equal across all producers, regardless of the risks of disease and of past and future claims emanating from employment therein? Would the tax be adequate to pay for the Trust Fund's obligations? And who would pay for claims filed in the early years of the program, where the last employment in the mines was after January 1, 1970? The latter problem arose because of two legislative changes in the 1977 amendments. First, coal mine operators previously had not been liable for claims filed prior to July 1, 1973 under the Part B program. Yet the 1977 changes made individual mine operators liable for claims filed at any time where coal mine employment had occurred prior to December 31, 1969. Congress had recast liability to be based not on the date of filing but on the date of last employment. Second, previously denied claims filed between January 1, 1970 and July 1, 1973 would have to be reconsidered by SSA and the Labor Department with more liberal criteria applied because of the 1977 amendments. Thus, denied claims that had once been the potential liability of the U.S. Treasury were to be reopened and could now become the liability of individual mine operators or, conceivably, their insurance carriers.

The trust fund concept satisfied those parties who wanted the coal mining industry, rather than the U.S. Treasury, to bear financial responsibility for black lung disease. Some involved parties would have preferred the Trust Fund to be used to pay for all successful claims, thereby eliminating individual mine operator liability. For example, Arnold Miller, President of the United Mine Workers of America, testified that this was his union's preference, primarily because it would remove the mine operators from the claims process.[3] The adversary process was perceived by the union to be responsible for many of the delays and claims denials that had characterized the Part C program.

The 1977 amendments meant that the Labor Department would dramatically alter its administration of black lung claims. First, it would now be able to award benefits to a larger proportion of claimants, including those previously denied claims that it would reassess. Second, it would have to develop procedures that would allow the Department to open the logjam that had developed, and to process incoming claims and deliver benefits more promptly. The 1977 amendments gave the agency the tools to carry out both of these goals. Subsequently, it would be argued that the Labor Department accomplished these goals at the expense of its compensating many claimants who were neither totally disabled due to pneumoconiosis nor survivors of miners who died from the disease. An alternative view was that, from 1978 to 1981, the Department responded to the clear call of the Congress in the 1977 amendments, much as SSA had emphatically responded to the 1972 amendments. As we will see, benefits during this period were awarded at a much higher approval rate than they had been, and the backlog was substantially reduced.

NOTES

1. *Legislative History of the Federal Coal Mine Health and Safety Act of 1969,* Part 2, prepared for the Subcommittee on Labor, U.S. Senate, 1975, p. 2117.

2. HR 3333.

3. Hearings before the Committee on Education and Labor, 95th Congress, 1st session, March 14-17, 1977.

• 3 •
Medical Issues
in Black Lung Compensation

In 1969, as members of both Houses of Congress debated the merits of Title IV of the Coal Mine Health and Safety Act, most appeared not to differentiate at all between terms such as black lung, pneumoconiosis, complicated pneumoconiosis, or some others that were bandied about. This may have reflected an inability on the part of some members to comprehend certain medical concepts or terminology, but it may also have been a sign of disinterest in an issue that promised to affect only small numbers of people and relatively few dollars. Yet major problems that soon surfaced in the program and continued to dog it over its entire existence were the product of this initial lack of precision. The focus of this chapter is on the medical issues that confronted the program.

While there were numerous difficult questions regarding the administration of this program, they all sprang from a single basic concept. It was the intent of Congress that a specific group of workers would be compensated if they had been rendered totally disabled due to a specific disease, or their survivors would be compensated if death was due to the specific disease. By limiting compensation to a specific population and a single disease, and by excluding partial disabilities for purposes of compensation, a set of very difficult decisions had to be made about how to construct the appropriate boundaries of the program. Since little or no

53

guidance was provided on these matters in the 1969 law, it was left originally to SSA to decide them. Dissatisfaction with that agency's administration was reflected in the passage of the 1972 amendments and, subsequently, the 1977 and 1981 amendments were products of congressional displeasure with the way that the boundaries were set by the Labor Department. A considerable amount of the blame for that displeasure, however, resulted from the ambiguities and vagueness in the legislation itself. What disease(s) did Congress seek to compensate? How was the disease to be identified? Did total disability mean what it had meant under the Social Security Disability Insurance program? Was the basis for compensation impairment or was it to be disability?

This chapter examines the three sets of medical issues that created intense controversy under the law. Each issue is treated separately here, but they are not entirely unrelated. The issues developed in the presence of scientific uncertainties, but not because a total lack of consensus or agreement existed. Instead, even where the medical-scientific community was largely, though not wholly, in agreement, the presence of any type of controversy enabled Congress to legislate without due consideration of the medical issues. The legislative branch sought to achieve certain social and economic goals and the existence of medical uncertainties or disputes enabled Congress to do precisely that.

The three sets of issues involve: (1) the methods appropriate to the diagnosis of the disease; (2) relating the presence of the disease to the assessment of disability; and (3) identifying the disease(s) to be compensated under law.[1] It is the third issue that is addressed here initially. Ironically, that issue had become relatively unimportant in most state workers' compensation laws, just as it grew controversial in the federal law. During the 1970s and 1980s, the states became generally less restrictive in their compensation for claims involving occupational diseases, ending the archaic practice of limiting compensation solely to diseases that were listed on a schedule. Had the states become more responsive to claimants with diseases prior to 1969, perhaps no black lung legislation would have developed. Yet, the perception that state practices had been and were restrictive led to passage of the 1969 law, which, ironically, itself was highly restrictive. It provided compensation to only a single class of occupational disease cases, black lung, and excluded all other diseases. In creating such a categoric entitlement, the law made the determination of black lung a critical component of the compensation process.

Coal Workers' Pneumoconiosis

Respiratory and pulmonary diseases among coal workers have long been known, if not well understood.[2] In 1831, Gregory identified coal as a factor in lung disease in miners. By 1837, Thomas Stratton had coined the name anthracosis. Until then, lung diseases in coal workers had been called miner's asthma. Observing lower death rates in miners than in other parts of the population, Smart wrote in 1885 that, "there must be some protective feature in coal mining operation, and that the preserving element might, after all, be the dust derived from the coal."[3] Indeed, this contributed to a view held by a number of physicians late in the 19th century and even into the early 20th century that coal dust had certain beneficial qualities for one's health. More likely, it probably reflected upon the good health of those who became coal miners.

Toward the end of the 19th century, mines in Great Britain became deeper and more machinery was introduced, with the consequence that more dust was produced and health conditions actually worsened. The increase in lung diseases in miners was believed by most authorities to be due to the free crystalline silica that was a by-product of the mining process. Whether silicosis or another form of dust-induced disease, that is, a pneumoconiosis, was responsible for the increase in lung disease remained to be established, but concern regarding the health of coal miners extended beyond Great Britain. Writing in 1925, H.R.M. Landis, a physician at the University of Pennsylvania, observed, "A man who works in a coal mine . . . sufficiently long will inevitably develop pneumonokoniosis [sic]. The changes may occur more quickly and be more extensive in one person than another . . . but there is no question as to the ultimate result. In fact, the progress of the pulmonary changes is so definite that, given the type of dust and the length of the exposure, one can almost predict the (X-ray) findings."[4]

A 1928 study by Collins and Gilchrist and another by Gough in 1940 appeared to establish that coal dust, in the absence of silica, could product pneumoconiosis. Autopsies confirmed the presence of disease without abnormal amounts of silica in the lungs.

A major watershed occurred when the Medical Research Council of Great Britain issued three separate reports on the subject in 1941, 1943, and 1945, which led directly to the placement of coal workers' pneumoconiosis on the schedule of compensable diseases. Indeed, the term coal workers' pneumoconiosis (CWP) first appeared in these reports. The British had found higher rates of CWP amongst anthracite miners, as well as differences related to the mines from which the coal was taken. At that time there was speculation that the chemical composition and the amount of volatile matter in the coal might explain some of these differences.

Research and interest in the U.S. in CWP lagged behind Britain. In the late 1950s and 1960s, several studies were done evaluating the causes of death among U.S. coal miners. Outside the research community, however, there appeared to be only limited recognition of the British findings that coal dust was associated with pneumoconiosis, aside from silicosis. It was only in the late 1960s and in the 1970s that coal workers' pneumoconiosis came to be recognized widely in this country as an occupational disease caused by coal dust.

The differentiation between silicosis and coal workers' pneumoconiosis was significant in both England and the U.S. Workers in most states and Great Britain who developed disabling silicosis could reasonably expect to receive some compensation for it, certainly by the late 1930s. However, if the symptoms of silicosis were not present or if the miner's work did not bring him into contact with silica, compensation was not likely to be paid. The symptoms of CWP and silicosis are not exactly alike. Consequently, miners would not be compensated in many instances where there was no silicosis present, though the worker was suffering from another pulmonary disorder which might have been CWP.

Coal workers' pneumoconiosis is a disorder caused by deposition of coal mine dust in the lungs.[5] It is customarily categorized into two sets: simple CWP and complicated CWP. According to a widely adopted scheme developed by and for the International Labor Organization and the University of Cincinnati, simple CWP is classified using the numbers 0, 1, 2, and 3. The patient is rated solely on the basis of X-rays, with the higher numbers indicative of larger numbers of small, pneumoconiotic opacities per unit area. A rating of 0 is indicative of few or no such opacities meaning the disease is not present. The rating 1 means few but definite opacities appear on the X-ray film and indicates that the disease is judged to be present, a 2 indicates the presence of a moderate number of small opacities and 3 is the classification when many small opacities are found. Within each numerical classification, a second number is added so that the rating can be further refined. Essentially, these second numbers connote below average, average, or above average within the major numerical categories.

While the major categories of simple CWP are classified by the numbers 1, 2, or 3, complicated CWP is classified by three letters, A, B, and C. Category A refers to the presence of one or more large opacities measuring one centimeter or more in diameter, with the sum total not exceeding five centimeters. Category B describes a greater involvement than A, and C defines a condition that is greater than B. In complicated pneumoconiosis, the large lesion that creates the opacity on the film is typically seen on a background with many small lesions characteristic of category 2 or 3 simple pneumoconiosis. A large lesion with no such background may indicate the presence of a tumor and no pneumoconiosis.

This system of classification, by itself, is not meant to explain the cause of the lesion(s) or to determine what type of pneumoconiosis, if any, is involved. Nor does the classification serve to describe the extent of respiratory impairment. X-ray findings similar to CWP could result from other conditions such as silicosis, berylliosis, aluminosis, talc pneumoconiosis or benign conditions like stannosis (tin) and silver polisher's lung.[6] However, this classification scheme has been useful beyond simply categorizing the extent of involvement as seen by the X-ray.

Most of the authorities on CWP use the term complicated CWP interchangeably with progressive massive fibrosis (PMF). At least one group has termed this imprecise,[7] but generally the two are treated as synonyms. This is the least of the problems of terminology. Testifying for the National Institute for Occupational Safety and Health on proposed federal regulations to administer the law, Dr. James Merchant observed, "There is still considerable confusion among U.S. pathologists as to what exactly constitutes

CWP. In addition, the terminology is confusing; an analysis of 1,300 cases submitted to the National Coal Miner Autopsy Study revealed that pathologists used 165 different terms to describe the lesion seen in coal workers' lungs. Currently, no pathological standards for CWP exist in the U.S."[8]

The ventilatory (or bellows) function of the lungs is measured by spirometry.[9] Evidence of impairment is associated with bronchitis, cigarette smoking and/or complicated CWP, but not with simple CWP. Persons with simple CWP are unaware of the presence of some impairment and usually become informed of the condition only after having been X-rayed. By contrast, persons with complicated CWP, particularly B or C, usually complain of shortness of breath (dyspnea) on exertion, and of coughing and sputum. Also, complicated CWP is associated with certain cardiopulmonary problems, including cor pulmonale (right ventricular disease and failure), that is not associated with simple CWP.

Coughing and sputum are found in many miners, but these symptons are equally likely to be present in miners with or without X-ray evidence of CWP. Where these conditions exist, they are typically due to (industrial) bronchitis or emphysema. This bronchitis, unlike that caused by cigarette smoking, has an insignificant clinical effect on ventilatory capacity.

The gas exchange function of the lungs shows a similar type of dichotomy between simple and complicated CWP. There is little or no deviation from the norm in miners with simple CWP. However, where complicated CWP, particularly category B or C is present, the diffusing capacity and the arterial blood gas tests reveal impairment, especially during exercise.

It is almost universally accepted that simple CWP (that is, categories 1, 2, or 3) is not disabling. Indeed, some individuals with simple CWP are unaware of any type of respiratory-pulmonary problems. Even less disagreement exists regarding the position that serious functional impairment is associated with category B or C of complicated CWP. As such, it is often disabling for persons employed in tasks involving some physical exertion. Some dispute exists on whether or not category A of complicated CWP virtually always causes serious functional impairment, as it does in category B or C.

Another significant difference between simple and complicated CWP is that the latter is considered to be progressive, in that it can advance even in the absence of further coal dust exposure. By contrast, simple CWP not only will not advance if exposure to coal dust ends, the condition can be reversed if the worker is removed from the hazardous exposure. Where workers with simple CWP continue to be exposed, their condition may advance so as to be classified as complicated CWP.

CWP rarely develops before 10 years of exposure to the dust. The incidence of CWP is higher among persons exposed to anthracite coal dust, a type of coal found only in this country in a small area of Pennsylvania and little mined in recent years. Its effects vary also by the region of the country where the coal is found, and also by the type of work done in the mines. The highest rates of simple CWP are found in Appalachia, the next highest in the Midwest and the lowest in the western part of the country. Simple CWP does not affect longevity. There is no effective treatment for complicated CWP but some forms of relief exist for the symptoms.

Another critical difference between simple and complicated CWP is the frequency with which they are found among active and former miners. Considerable evidence exists regarding the differential incidence of simple and complicated CWP among miner populations. While there are some significant differences reported among different studies, it is absolutely clear that complicated CWP tends to be found relatively infrequently compared to simple CWP. The differences in findings by medical researchers as to the relative occurrence of simple and complicated CWP likely derive from differences in populations being examined. In one study 9,706 miners from 21 bituminous mines and 2 anthracite mines were examined between 1969 and 1971.[10] W. Keith Morgan found almost 30 percent had simple CWP and about 2.5 percent had PMF. (Many of the latter cases came from the anthracite mines.) Roger Mitchell estimated that 10 percent-30 percent of current miners have CWP with perhaps one-third of these having PMF.[11] He cited further evidence from Great Britain that about 1 percent of simple CWP cases become complicated each year. Earlier in the same report, it is estimated that 2 percent of simple CWP cases a year become complicated CWP.[12] About 70 percent of those persons with complicated CWP are in category A, where there is less likelihood of serious functional impairment than in categories B and C.

During the 1970s, NIOSH began an extensive program to monitor the health of coal miners, providing additional evidence on the incidence of CWP. Data from two of their recent surveys, presented in table 3.1, indicated lower levels of CWP, and especially of complicated pneumoconiosis, than do the studies cited earlier. Aside from some differences in research methodologies, the different findings of these later studies may be explained, in part at least, by two phenomena. First, persons with CWP may have dropped out of coal mining and are no longer in the group surveyed, due to the presence of the Black Lung programs. Second, the dust controls imposed by the 1969 legislation may account for some of the apparent decline in incidence. It is unlikely, however, that these controls could have had a major impact on PMF, particularly in the Round Two Surveillance Study (see table 3.1), since it was undertaken from mid-1973 to early 1975.

The differences between simple and complicated CWP described above place the 1969 legislative debate into somewhat better perspective. The version of the bill that finally passed the House of Representatives (HR 13950), provided compensation specifically for "complicated pneumoconiosis," which was defined precisely in section 110(b) (7) (B): "The term 'complicated pneumoconiosis' means an advanced stage of a chronic coal dust of the lung which (i) when diagnosed by chest roentgenogram yields one or more large opacities (greater than one centimeter in diameter) and would be classified in Category A, B, or C in the International Classification . . . by the International Labor Organization. . . ." Had this language been retained it would have ruled out compensation for the far larger cohort of miners or former miners with simple CWP or other pulmonary-respiratory diseases. Moreover, it would have made the process of identifying eligible claimants much simpler than it eventually was, since category A, B, or C is not difficult to observe by trained roentgenologists. The Senate's version of the 1969 law also limited benefits to persons with "complicated pneumoconiosis" from coal mine employment. While that bill provided no definition of complicated pneumoconiosis, there has been no controversy over either the meaning of complicated pneumoconiosis or its diagnosis.

Although both the House and the Senate bills specifically limited compensation to complicated CWP, the term "complicated" had been dropped when the bill emerged from the Conference Committee. In section 402(b), the law defined pneumoconiosis as "a chronic dust disease of the lung arising out of employment in an underground coal mine." By entirely eliminating the term "complicated" that had ap-

Table 3.1
Coal Workers' Pneumoconiosis—The NIOSH National Coal Workers' Health Surveillance Program

Round Two (1973-1975)

Years mining	Total # miners	Radiographic category (ILO-U/C) (Percent)				
		0	1	2	3	PMF
0 to 9	91,159	99.3	0.6	0.0	0.0	0.0
10 to 19	8,398	87.1	11.6	1.0	0.1	0.3
20 to 29	7,609	72.2	21.5	5.1	0.3	0.9
30 to 39	5,392	62.0	27.3	8.0	1.2	1.6
40 plus	1,615	56.0	30.2	9.2	1.2	3.5
Total	114,173	94.2	4.5	0.9	0.1	0.2

Round Three (1978-1980)

Years mining	Total # miners	Radiographic category (ILO-U/C) (Percent)				
		0	1	2	3	PMF
0 to 9	39,483	98.9	1.1	0.0	0.0	0.0
10 to 19	6,618	93.2	6.4	0.3	0.2	0.1
20 to 29	2,704	82.4	15.2	1.9	0.2	0.3
30 to 39	2,919	71.7	21.5	4.5	0.3	2.0
40 plus	554	66.6	24.4	5.8	0.7	2.5
Total	52,278	95.5	3.9	0.5	0.4	0.2

SOURCE: Summary tables appear in materials prepared by NIOSH, Hearings before the Subcommittee on Oversight of the Committee on Ways and Means, House of Representatives, July 27, September 28, 1981, p. 32.

peared in both the Senate and House bills, and by an immense revision of the definition from the version originally passed by the House, the Conference Committee was able to completely alter the character of the law.

The disease(s) to be compensated under the 1969 law had been described as pneumoconiosis or PMF and not as "black lung." With one or two exceptions, the term "black lung" does not appear in the scientific literature until 1969 or shortly thereafter. There is a medical condition, anthracosis, which refers to the blackening of the lungs found in coal miners. By 1920, however, it was realized that this was merely a pigment deposition, found widely at autopsy in persons from industrialized areas far removed from coal mining regions, and not a disease. Thus, the term used in 1969 and thereafter, black lung, is a legal or political concept and not a medical one. As such, it applies to whatever disease(s) the lawmakers or administrators wish it to. Unlike the fairly precise medical meaning of simple or complicated CWP, the term black lung has the twin virtues to some of being catchy and emotional, while providing maximum flexibility or ambiguity.

The term, black lung, did not appear in either the House or Senate version of the 1969 law, but is found in the bill reported by the Conference Committee. While it is not used in the text of the various sections of the law, Title IV is entitled "Black Lung Benefits."

By defining pneumoconiosis as it did, and by using the term black lung rather than CWP, the law opened the door to claims for a variety of respiratory and pulmonary diseases that are not CWP. It also created a variety of problems for those charged with administering the program. First, it raised expectations among miners, their families and their representatives that compensation would be forthcoming for virtually all pulmonary-respiratory diseases contracted by a miner, not simply for a single, reasonably well-defined one. Second, partly because of the original language in the separate Senate and House bills, many persons believed that only CWP was to be compensable under the law. That notion was reinforced by the language in the law which referred to "pneumoconiosis." Third, the definition of the disease that was inserted by the Conference Committee forced the law's administrators to identify those other diseases and conditions that would be compensable on the grounds that they arise out of coal mine employment and are dust-induced.

Aside from CWP, at least two other lung conditions are understood to be related to coal mining. Silicosis (another type of pneumoconiosis) is found in workers involved in mine construction or transportation work.[13] These workers are exposed to aerosolized sands applied to the rail tracks in the mines to provide some traction. Construction workers, primarily roof bolters, also are exposed when they bore holes in the rock strata outside the coal seam. Generally, the presence of the disease is diagnosed by X-ray.

The other lung disease that is widely associated with coal mining is industrial bronchitis. Workers in all dusty trades can develop industrial bronchitis, which results from the dust being deposited in the trachea and bronchi, the airways that carry the inhaled air to the gas-exchanging portion of the lung. A properly functioning lung performs two necessary functions. First, it acts as a bellows, moving both inhaled air into the lungs and exhaled air out of the body. Second, the gas exchange function occurs as oxygen is transferred to the blood and carbon dioxide is removed from it to be exhaled. Dust in the trachea and bronchi may reduce the ventilatory capacity (the bellows function) of the patient, but not substantially. The body seeks to rid itself of the dust particles by producing excess mucus, leading to phlegm and coughing. Because the particles are removed, the condition does not appear on X-rays.

The presence of coughing and sputum and slight reductions in ventilatory capacity occur no more frequently in miners with simple CWP than in those without the condition. Increasing the degree of simple CWP (and thereby the dust content of the lungs) does not lead to concomitant reductions in ventilatory capacity. Miners with reduced ventilatory function have difficulty due to the obstruction of the airways reflecting industrial bronchitis, and not due to simple CWP. Obstructed airways due to coal dust may be uncomfortable but are not likely to cause disability. However, for persons with PMF, more serious airway obstruction may exist, and consequently substantial functional impairment may be present. The incidence of breathing impairments in coal miners is significant. The National Study of Coal Workers' Pneumoconiosis surveyed the health condition of over 9,300 miners. It reported that 40.4 percent suffered some form of bronchitis, 11.2 percent had persistent breathlessness, and 24.2 percent had "significant" airway obstruction.[14]

Cigarette smoking is also a cause of obstructed airways. Unlike industrial bronchitis, however, cigarette smoking is associated with a loss of flexibility in the lungs (emphysema) and destroys their ability to exchange gas. There does not appear to be any special synergism between cigarette smoking and coal dust, however, as in the case of asbestos exposure. In miners with chronically obstructed airways, the relative contributory causes as apportioned between cigarette smoking and coal mine dust are a matter of dispute. The director of NIOSH has suggested that about 50 percent of the cases arising in coal miners are due to cigarettes.[15] Dr. W. Keith Morgan directly challenged this estimate. Based on comparisons of nonsmoking surface miners with nonsmoking mine face employees, he found that the average ventilatory capacities were 102 percent and 98 percent, respectively, of the predicted normal values. He termed this difference "statistically significant" but "clinically insignificant."[16] Based on this he assessed cigarette smoking as having from 6 to 10 times the effect of coal dust on ventilatory capacity.

The product of these legislative ambiguities and medical uncertainties were administrative, political and informational problems. In the first two-three years under the new law, numerous claims were denied to severely impaired miners, former miners or survivors of workers who had respiratory and pulmonary conditions at the time of their death. The basis for the denials tended to be X-rays that displayed no evidence of disabling pneumoconiosis. Some of these people suffered "black lung," however, to the extent that they did have industrial bronchitis, or cigarette-induced bronchitis and emphysema. Denials of compensation benefits by the Social Security Administration infuriated the supporters of the black lung program in Congress, the United Mine Workers union and the various Black Lung Associations. The key source of the problem, however, was the ambiguity created by the 1969 law regarding the disease(s) to be compensated. Reflecting this, Senator Byrd of West Virginia argued, "Let us stop quibbling with dying men as to whether their lungs are riddled with black lung or whether they are afflicted with asthma, or silicosis, or chronic bronchitis."[17]

Congress took three steps to force the Social Security Administration and the Labor Department to widen the coverage of the law beyond CWP. In the 1972 amendments it moved indirectly by disallowing X-ray evidence as the sole basis for denial of a claim. Thus, persons with no evidence of CWP based on X-rays were now to be eligible for benefits.

Second, it added the 15-year rule (section 411(c)): a rebuttable presumption of pneumoconiosis was established retroactive to December 30, 1969, for a coal miner who worked 15 years in underground mines (or in substantially similar conditions), if the person had a totally disabling pulmonary or respiratory condition, even with a chest X-ray that was negative for pneumoconiosis. The presumption clearly smoothed the path of claimants unable to demonstrate CWP due to negative X-rays.

Finally, in the 1977 amendments, Congress reworded its 1969 definition of pneumoconiosis so as to make it far more inclusive: "The term 'pneumoconiosis' means a chronic dust disease of the lung *and its sequela, including respiratory and pulmonary impairments,* arising out of coal mine employment."[18] (The underlined words were those added by the 1977 amendments.) While scientists could be left to ponder and argue what this meant, the intent of Congress to widen the basis of eligibility was absolutely clear to the administrators of the program. The disease(s) to be covered under the law was (were) much more than CWP.

The meaning of the disease(s) to be compensated was not settled with the 1977 amendments. In April 1978, the Department of Labor issued proposed regulations to implement the 1977 amendments. Included was an elaboration of the definition of pneumoconiosis.[19] Almost two years later, the final version of the Department's regulations implementing the amendments of 1977 was issued.[20] In the Labor Department's interpretation, the definition ". . . includes, but is not limited to, coal workers' pneumoconiosis, anthracosilicosis, anthracosis, massive pulmonary fibrosis, progressive massive fibrosis, silicosis or silicotuberculosis, arising out of coal mine employment. For purposes of this definition, a disease 'arising out of coal mine employment' *includes any chronic pulmonary disease resulting in respiratory or pulmonary impairment significantly related to, or substantially aggravated by, dust exposure in coal mine employment.*"[21] (Italics added here for emphasis.) In issuing its proposed regulations in 1978, the Labor Department had proposed to explicitly exclude lung cancer and diseases of bacteriological or viral origin from being considered to have arisen out of dust exposure in coal mine employment. One measure of the Department's timidity in the face of oversight by Rep. Perkins and other advocates of a more liberalized program was that it backed off from even this in its final version. It chose not to specify bronchitis and emphysema as chronic pulmonary diseases that arise out of coal mine employment. However, since the interpretation of the definition was not limited to the diseases listed, bronchitis and emphysema were clearly compensable, so long as other criteria for benefits were also met.

The Labor Department also sought as inclusive a definition as possible through the use of the aggravation theory. Under the Department's regulation, a claimant need only show that dust exposure in coal mine employment substantially aggravated an underlying or pre-existing condition. Indeed this was somewhat stricter than the regulations proposed in 1978 which did not include the word "substantially." This tightening probably resulted from a hint provided by the courts after the proposed regulations were issued that the Department may have overstepped its legislative grounds in interpreting the meaning of pneumoconiosis in this way.[22]

To summarize, coal workers' pneumoconiosis is a discrete disease, now recognized as such by the medical community. In its simple form, the condition is not disabling. In 1969, both Houses of Congress endorsed a new entitlements program for workers disabled by or deceased due to complicated CWP. The Conference Committee eliminated the term "complicated," and defined somewhat vaguely the disease to be compensated. The definition was modified in 1977 to permit broader coverage. The Labor Department, eager to overcome its inability to compensate most applicants, further extended the disease(s) to be compensated through the regulations it issued in 1978 and 1980. By then, "black lung" bore little relationship to coal workers' pneumoconiosis.

Diagnosis

The expressed aim of Congress in 1969 was to compensate coal miners totally disabled or killed due to pneumoconiosis arising out of underground coal mine employment. Had Congress meant to compensate only complicated CWP, or even CWP (in the presence of functional impairment), the matter of diagnosis would have been relatively straightforward. As noted earier in this chapter, the presence or absence of pneumoconiosis can be found by qualified readers of chest X-rays where the film quality is adequate. While X-ray evidence does not completely simplify an adjudicator's needs where only pneumoconiosis is to be compensable, it makes the task quite manageable.

If one has a compensation program dealing solely with disability or death due to CWP, there are at least five diagnostic problems that exist where X-ray films are used as the primary method of screening or diagnosis. One type of problem exists where one or more large (1 cm. or larger in diameter) lesions appear on X-rays. Though this is characteristic of complicated CWP, it may also be evidence of other diseases, including some other pneumoconioses such as silicosis. X-ray evidence is problematic where silicosis is not compensable but CWP is. The matter can be dealt with, though not to the satisfaction of all parties, by using presumptions involving work histories. Large lesions may also be seen in X-rays where a tumor is present. However, complicated CWP, as distinct from a tumor, is typically characterized by a large lesion or lesions on a background consistent with category 2 or 3 pneumoconiosis. Thus, the presence of large lesions can usually be diagnosed correctly as pneumoconiosis or not.

A more difficult problem occurs at the very margin of category 1 (simple) pneumoconiosis and category 0 (no pneumoconiosis).[23] where the presence of pneumoconiosis is a necessary condition for compensation, difficulties can occur due to challenges in diagnosing the presence of the disease at its very earliest stages. This is complicated by the fact that some opacities that appear in chest X-rays may be related solely to the aging process. Dr. Russell Morgan has written, "The problem here is that pneumoconiosis is not the only condition that manifests itself by the presence of small, rounded or irregular opacities on the chest roentgenogram. Many other states, including some that might be considered to be normal physiological processes (e.g., aging) may produce them too."[24]

A third set of problems occurs because the quality of the film may affect the ability to make a diagnosis or may affect the finding itself. One authority estimates that perhaps 25 percent of the roughly 20,000 X-rays he has read of workers who have been occupationally exposed to various dusts were of substandard diagnostic quality, or unreadable for purposes of detecting and classifying pneumoconiosis.[25] Where the film is underexposed, the less experienced reader will have a tendency to find disease where none is present. Where the X-ray film is overexposed it can cause the changes due to pneumoconiosis to be masked or obliterated. Morgan also pointed to the problem of poor quality X-rays for purposes of proper diagnosis.[26]

A related but separate issue that created immense difficulties under the law is the technical ability of X-ray readers. Even where the quality of X-ray films is satisfactory, not all physicians possess the skill or the training to properly read them. Testifying in 1978, Dr. William Cole estimated that "less than 200 physicians and radiologists have demonstrated a proficiency in the correct use of the classifications system" (the ILO-U/C scheme).[27]

The need for expert readers of X-ray films became apparent early in the life of the black lung program. In 1976, NIOSH, in association with the Johns Hopkins School of Medicine, developed an examination to test the proficiency of readers in classifying chest roentgenograms. Of the first 140 persons to take the examination, 77 were passed, thereby, qualifying as "B" readers. These experts worked as consultants to the government and were used to review X-rays and findings sent in from the field. An "A" reader is typically a local physician who has taken a course directed by NIOSH/Johns Hopkins or has otherwise demonstrated a proficiency in the ILO-U/C system. "B" readers have demonstrated a higher level of proficiency than "A" readers.

The issues of film and reader quality have been posed here in the abstract. In fact, the U.S. Department of Labor conducted a study in 1977 where its expert "B" readers evaluated 18,014 X-rays and the reports filed on them by the field physicians who had evaluated black lung claims for the Department. (See table 3.2 below.) The study demonstrated a widespread pattern of disparities with a strong bias toward field physicians finding excessive (unwarranted) instances of disease. For example, and at its worst, the study found that in 10,044 instances where field physicians reported finding simple pneumoconiosis, over 10 percent of the X-rays were unreadable. Of the balance of almost 9,000 cases, only 27.5 percent were actually simple pneumoconiosis, according to expert readers. Over 70 percent were judged to be not pneumoconiosis, and 2.4 percent were found to be complicated pneumoconiosis.

The problem of X-ray reader quality stems from several underlying causes. At one level, the ability to read such X-rays properly develops with experience. Moreover, the skill will atrophy if not maintained. At another level, some physicians have a reputation as being more or less inclined to find pneumoconiosis. In the coal mining areas, some physicians developed reputations as being "sympathetic" to miners and were prone to diagnose pneumoconiosis. Some doctors had precisely the opposite reputation. Testifying in 1981, Dr. Keith Morgan argued "I regret that many radiologists invariably interpret every film as positive. In the case of certain radiologists whose services are invariably given to claimants, I have yet to see an X-ray which has not been read as positive. In looking through a hundred consecutive reports of one of these radiologists, all of which were reported as either category 2 or 3 simple CWP, only seven were subsequently reported as positive by a 'B' reader."[28]

Aside from the issues noted, X-rays have other limitations as a means of screening workers for compensation benefits. Clearly, mechanisms must be developed to determine compensability where claimants have died without having chest X-rays prior to death. Further, X-rays can indicate the presence of disease but not necessarily the degree of functional impairment. The matter can be partially finessed, as in the case of black lung, by creating the presumption in the law that complicated pneumoconiosis was totally disabling. However, for the far more common cases involving the radiological diagnosis of simple pneumoconiosis, other criteria must be developed to measure impairment/disability and determine eligibility for compensation.

The shortcomings and limitations of X-ray evidence in pneumoconiosis claims make several other methods of diagnosis useful. For example, autopsies are considered a highly effective way of establishing that the deceased person had CWP at the time of death. It is also useful in establishing the cause of death and the linkages between the pulmonary-respiratory disease and any other factors causing death. The

Table 3.2
Comparative Results of readings by Field Physicians and "B" Readers
Identifying 18,014 Chest Roentgenograms for the Department of Labor in 1977

1. # of films classified negative by field physicians — 7603
    less # of films declared unreadable by "B" readers — 668
    # of readable films classified negative by field physicians — 6935
    # of these films classified negative by "B" readers — 6299 or 90.8%
    # of these films upgraded to simple pneumoconiosis by "B" readers — 609 or 8.8%
    # of these films upgraded to complicated pneumoconiosis by "B" readers — 27 or 0.4%

2. # of films classified simple pneumoconiosis by field physicians — 10044
    less # of films declared unreadable by "B" readers — 1049
    # of readable films classified by simple pneumoconiosis by "B" readers — 2570 or 27.5%
    # of these films downgraded to negative by "B" readers — 6304 or 70.1%
    # of these films upgraded to complicated by "B" readers — 221 or 2.4%

3. # of films classified complicated pneumoconiosis by field physicians — 367
    less # of films declared unreadable by "B" readers — 29
    # of readable films classified complicated pneumoconiosis by field physicians — 338
    # of these films classified complicated pneumoconiosis by "B" readers — 120 or 35.5%
    # of these films downgraded to negative by "B" readers — 123 or 36.4%
    # of these films downgraded to simple pneumoconiosis by "B" readers — 95 or 28.1%

4.	# of films classified negative by "B" readers	12716
	# of these films classified negative by field physicians	6299 or 49.5%
	# of these films upgraded to simple pneumoconiosis by field physicians	6304 or 49.5%
	# of these films upgraded to complicated pneumoconiosis by field physicians	123 or 1.0%
5.	# of films classified simple pneumoconiosis by "B" readers	3174
	# of these films classified simple pneumoconiosis by field physicians	2470 or 77.8%
	# of these films downgraded to negative by field physicians	609 or 19.2%
	# of these films upgraded to complicated pneumoconiosis by field physicians	95 or 3.0%
6.	# of cases classified complicated pneumoconiosis by "B" readers	368
	# of these cases classified complicated pneumoconiosis by field physicians	120 or 32.6%
	# of these cases downgraded to negative by field physicians	27 or 7.3%
	# of these cases downgraded to simple pneumoconiosis by field physicians	221 or 60.1%

SOURCE: Department of Labor.

1969 act mandated the National Coal Workers' Autopsy Study, which provided a voluntary, cost-free autopsy for any former underground miner.

Dr. James Merchant of NIOSH testified on certain findings from the National Coal Workers' Autopsy Study which matched the autopsy findings with the death certificates prepared by the worker's local physician.[29] Based on 1,300 cases from 1970 to 1974, NIOSH reported that of the major disease categories found to be the *underlying* cause of death, e.g., lung cancer, tuberculosis, chronic obstructive airway disease, heart disease, 10 to 30 percent were not shown on the death certificate. Where autopsy revealed these diseases to be a *contributing* cause of death, they were not found on death certificates in over 50 percent of the cases. The study confirmed the fallibility of relying too heavily on death certificates for compensation purposes (or for that matter for epidemiological work), and the desirability of using autopsy as a diagnostic tool.

In practice, autopsy evidence was treated as having essential limitations under this program. That is most clearly reflected by the Labor Department's rules: "Because of the nature of autopsy, autopsy findings are accorded a high probative value. However, the claims examiner must keep in mind that the physician normally applies a narrow, scientific or medical definition of pneumoconiosis, while the claims examiner uses a broader, legal definition. Interpretation of autopsy reports is further complicated by the absence of any widely agreed-upon standards for the diagnosis of pneumoconiosis on autopsy, or for classification of the stage of advancement."[30]

Aside from X-rays and autopsy, pneumoconiosis can be also detected by the use of biopsy. Bits of lung tissue are removed and examined either during surgical procedures or by inserting a needle and removing such small pieces. The latter is widely regarded as involving some risk to the patient, and is therefore widely considered inappropriate for use solely in the diagnosis for compensation purposes.

If the disease to be compensated was exclusively CWP, particularly complicated CWP, the means to make proper diagnosis would have been available readily to program administrators since 1970. Obviously, the core problem was that it was black lung and not CWP that Congress wanted to compensate. Whatever was meant by the "legal disease" black lung, its diagnosis was far less clear than that of CWP. By extending the disease definition well beyond CWP, the law eventually forced program administrators to work in the roundabout way of establishing, first, the existence of an impairment, and then using that to establish the presence of the compensable disease.

While the 1969 law was ambiguous, at best, in identifying the compensable disease, the agency charged with administering the law initially was confronted with the task of determining eligibility in actual cases. Based on the Social Security Administration's reading of the law, the agency opted to compensate pneumoconiosis (as the law stated) and not the medically undefined disease(s) "black lung," as the law also stated. The criteria employed by SSA were straightforward and partially relied on SSA's experience in evaluating total disability under section 223 of the Social Security Act. In its defense, SSA was given virtually no opportunity to fully explore criteria for determining compensability. Incredibly, the 1969 law mandated that HEW promulgate its regulations for determining total disability and death due to pneumoconiosis by the end of the third month following the month of enactment. The agency published its regulations in the Federal Register and made them effective immediately. While it invited the public to comment on these regulations and to submit data and arguments about them, ultimately the agency did not change its regulations until forced to do so by the 1972 amendments. To be sure, the agency was experienced in operating a total disability insurance program, but it acknowledged that it had not administered a program where eligibility was based on disability due to a specific disease only, and where a causal connection had to be established with a specific type of employment (underground coal mining).

Initially, SSA operated under relatively simple decision rules. Where X-rays revealed the presence of complicated CWP, section 411(b) (3) created the irrebuttable presumption of total disability or death due to pneumoconiosis. Where X-rays revealed no pneumoconiosis, the claim was denied. This decision reflected the medical concept of the disease, CWP, and not the "legal disease" that black lung could have implied.

> To establish the causal or occupational connection with coal workers' pneumoconiosis, the regulations provide that there must be X-ray evidence of pneumoconiosis in the living applicant (in a rare case, a biopsy). This is based on the prevailing medical judgement that in the absence of positive X-ray evidence, the disease does not exist or exists to a degree that would have no significant effect on the claimant's functional capacity.

> There is some minority medical opinion to the effect that disabling pneumoconiosis may exist in the absence of "positive" X-ray evidence thereof. However, this issue was thoroughly considered by the Social Security Administration, through extensive consultation with a wide range of medical specialists, and the requirement was included in the regulations as reflecting the overwhelming consensus of medical judgement on the issue.[31]

What remained for SSA was the very considerable task of dealing with claimants who were found to have simple pneumoconiosis. Section 413(b) of the statute required the agency to make entitlement determinations "to the maximum extent feasible" according to the procedures used in the Social Security Disability Insurance program. Thus, in the presence of simple CWP the claimant's ventilatory functioning was tested and standards were adopted that were basically the same as those already in place in the disability insurance program. Indeed, the agency argued that, in the presence of uncertainty, its administration of the program erred on the side of generosity:

> An individual's ventilatory ability may be compromised by many diseases other than coal workers' pneumoconiosis. Emphysema commonly affects this ability: neurological, muscular, infectious, or degenerative disease may do so also. From a medical standpoint, it is impossible in most situations to determine what portion of an individual's reduced ventilatory capacity is due to coal workers' pneumoconiosis and what portion is due to one or more other diseases he has. Nevertheless, to assure fullest equity to claimants under these circumstances, favorable disability determinations have been made where a claimant has a serious breathing impairment and has pneumoconiosis.[32]

The implication of this admitted practice was that diagnosis followed from the finding of impairment, given any evidence of the presence of simple CWP, no matter how early or limited the stage.

SSA drew the line where no evidence of pneumoconiosis was found. "Some miners have emphysema or chronic bronchitis and may be severely disabled as a result, but do not have pneumoconiosis. Under the law, claims from such

miners   must   be   denied.''[33]   No   doubt,   the   agency's
understanding of the law followed from the language making compensation limited to pneumoconiosis.

SSA's treatment of death claims paralleled that employed
for living miners except where the 411(c) (2) presumption required otherwise. That provision presumed death due to
pneumoconiosis when a person employed 10 years or more in
underground mining died of a "respiratory disease." Sec.
411(c) (3) created the irrebuttable presumption that death
was due to pneumoconiosis (regardless of actual cause)
where the miner had had complicated pneumoconiosis.
Where the miner did not have complicated pneumoconiosis,
and where 411(c) (2) did not apply, the agency could and did
find grounds for compensation where respiratory disease
may have contributed to the deceased miner's demise.
"Unless death is due to trauma or clearly results from an
acute disease process, the Social Security Administration has
ordinarily held that pneumoconiosis or 'respirable disease,'
if present, was a significant contributing factor in causing
death."[34]

According to SSA, most of the death claims that were
denied were characterized in either of two ways. In some
claims, there was no evidence of chronic lung disease. In
others, the miner died either from an acute disease unrelated
to pneumoconiosis or from trauma where complicated
pneumoconiosis was not found.

The presumption under 411(c) (2), which provided
benefits where death was due to "respirable" disease rather
than pneumoconiosis, was justified by its proponents on
several grounds. First, many U.S. doctors had never
recognized CWP as a disease until recently. Widows would
have been hard pressed to win claims without such a
presumption since death certificates or medical reports
would have otherwise undermined their chances for benefits.

Also, since hard medical evidence would be difficult to obtain where deaths had occurred in earlier years, the standard of proof was eased. Since the presumption was rebuttable where medical evidence did exist and where the worker died in the absence of complicated CWP, SSA could have sought to rebut the presumption when another respirable disease was the cause of death. Apparently, this was infrequently or never done.

Despite what appeared to be a magnanimous approach to claimants, SSA received immense criticism for its administration of the act from the law's strongest supporters. By December 31, 1971, more claims had been denied than were allowed (163,000 denials compared to 159,000 allowed).[35] Miners, their representatives, and others could point to denials in cases where former miners with lung impairments were barely ambulatory, side by side with allowed claims where men still worked in mines. (The latter were workers whose X-rays showed the presence of complicated CWP, and who gained entitlement through the irrebuttable presumption found in sec. 411(b) (3).) The hearings that preceded the 1972 amendments were filled with criticism of SSA officials. Considerable anger was expressed at the negative presumption applied by SSA, which found miners ineligible for benefits where there was no X-ray evidence of pneumoconiosis.

A reading of the hearings and the floor debates that preceded the 1972 amendments provides a classic illustration of the adversaries' inability to communicate with each other. Black lung supporters insisted that SSA had denied large numbers of worthy claimants with serious lung diseases because of the agency's insistence that X-rays show signs of the disease. They assembled some evidence from the medical community, depending heavily on Dr. Donald L. Rasmussen, that concluded that *black lung* could exist in the

absence of positive X-ray evidence. Led by Rep. John Erlenborn, opponents argued that *coal workers' pneumoconiosis*
was detectable by X-ray and that no better, single method existed to diagnose the disease. Responding to the charge by
supporters of a more generous program that CWP or
fibrosis had been found on autopsy of the lungs of miners
who had been denied benefits, opponents argued that early
stages of simple CWP could have been present, but that this
would hardly have caused impairment or death.

One interpretation of the debate is that serious technical
and definitional issues were present and that many members
of Congress could not understand them. Even if that view is
correct for most of the members, the issues were clearly not
beyond the grasp of Congressmen Perkins and Erlenborn.
Their substantial quarrel was a repeat of the bitter differences that emerged over the original Conference Committee's revision that changed "complicated coal workers'
pneumoconiosis" to "pneumoconiosis" and to "black
lung." Lurking behind this fundamental difference was the
extent to which this program conferred very broad or narrow
eligibility to entitlements to older miners and their survivors.

The heated nature of the debate did not reflect the relative
strength of the adversaries. A key vote in the House on a
measure proposed by Erlenborn to stop the bill, failed on a
voice vote, and the House bill was passed 311-79, with 40
members not voting. The Senate version of the bill was passed unanimously.

For purposes of widening the scope of eligibility for
benefits in the 1972 amendments, two key measures were
taken. First, sec. 413 was amended to add the following:

> . . . no claim for benefits under this part shall be
> denied solely on the basis of the results of a chest
> roentgenogram. In determining the validity of
> claims under this part (part B), all relevant evidence

shall be considered, including where relevant, medical tests such as blood gas studies, X-ray examination, electrocardiogram, pulmonary function studies, or physical performance tests, and any medical history, evidence submitted by the claimant's physician or his wife's affidavits and in case of a deceased miner, other appropriate affidavits of persons with knowledge of the miner's physical condition, and other supportive material.

Thus, Congress made its will clear to SSA. The diagnostic standards for determining the presence of black lung were to be loosened, most directly by eliminating the screening device of the X-ray. By adding a list of other medical evidence to be considered, and in the context of the evident dissatisfaction with the large numbers of rejections of claims, Congress told SSA to find ways to justify compensating claimants. Just so that was clear to SSA, the Senate's Committee on Labor and Public Welfare explained its intent: "It is not the Committee's intention that all of these types of evidence be secured in every claim but that such evidence be sought in those claims as is necessary *to assure a decision on the claim consistent with the remedial nature of the legislation* (italics added by the author).[36]

The other method used by Congress to widen the eligibility boundaries of the program was less obvious than the section 413 amendment but no less subtle. When Senator Randolph's report of the committee's bill emerged, it contained the following:

The backlog of claims which have been filed under these provisions cannot await the establishment of new facilities or the development of new medical procedures. They must be handled under present circumstances in the light of limited medical resources and techniques.

> Accordingly the Committee expects the Secretary
> to adopt such interim evidentiary rules and disabili-
> ty evaluation criteria as will permit prompt and
> vigorous processing of the large backlog of claims
> consistent with the language and intent of these
> amendments. Such interim rules and criteria shall
> give full consideration to the combined employ-
> ment handicap of disease and age. . . .[37]

It is striking that no comparable statement appears in the
report of the Committee on Education and Labor in the
House of Representatives,[38] nor was there any such reference
in the legislation itself. Yet the committee's sentiments were
well understood, particularly in the context of the amendments and the one-sided votes that supported them. Mark
Solomons argues that the statement in the Senate report was
conceived by HEW officials and Senate staff "as a convenient mechanism to permit the adoption of temporary rules
to expedite the approval of a much large number of
claims."[39]

The arrangement was created and rationalized on the
grounds that adequate medical facilities were not in place to
properly diagnose and evaluate the many black lung
claimants, including those whose claims had been denied
previously by SSA and would now be reopened due to the
1972 amendments. To expedite the process of cutting into
the backlog, "interim criteria" were to be created by SSA
and applied to Part B claimants. "Permanent criteria"
which were essentially those used by SSA since 1970 would
be used by the Department of Labor to administer the Part C
program when it eventually took over the administration of
new claims on July 1, 1973. By that time, it was presumed
that better exercise or physical performance testing facilities
would be widely available in coal mining areas. More important, the mine operators would have to take financial responsibility for the Part C program.

The interim criteria (also called the interim presumptions) were proposed by SSA on September 2, 1972 in a Notice of Rule Making published in the *Federal Register,* with interested parties given only until September 20, 1972 to submit comments. On September 30, 1972, the regulations for the interim and permanent criteria were published in final form in the *Federal Register.*[40]

SSA paraphrased the language of the Senate Committee's report in explaining why it developed the interim criteria.[41] However, SSA described itself as fulfilling "congressional intent" when indeed it was actually responding to a statement in a committee report, without explicit legislative support.[42]

The interim presumptions greatly eased the burden of claimants by substantially lowering the criteria for eligibility. First, they created a rebuttable presumption of total disability due to pneumoconiosis where X-ray evidence showed the presence of simple pneumoconiosis *or* where ventilatory function studies demonstrated the presence of chronic disabling pulmonary or respiratory disease and the claimant had worked 10 years or more in coal mine employment. The interim criteria allowed benefits either solely on the basis of an X-ray or ventilatory tests. SSA acknowledged that the crucial ventilatory criteria were more liberal than those in the permanent criteria. The reason given for this was that these more liberal criteria would compensate somewhat for the inability of SSA to identify workers with impaired diffusion capacity, that is, the ability to transfer oxygen efficiently from the lungs to the blood. Such tests could not be carried out due to a lack of testing facilities or sometimes because claimants were physically unable to perform the exercise part of a test of diffusion capacity.

The ventilatory function tests were tied to the rebuttable presumption that disability or death was due to pneumoconiosis arising out of coal mine employment if the tests indicated impairment, and the miner had been employed 10 years or more in underground (or, with comparable conditions, surface) coal mining. The presumption could be rebutted if the miner was still employed in his usual coal mining work or in comparable and gainful employment. Conceivably, it could also be rebutted if other physical tests indicated that no impairment was present

The interim presumptions meant that SSA had developed an entirely new perception of congressional intent after the 1972 amendments. Essentially, where virtually any evidence of pulmonary or respiratory impairment was found, the claim was paid. Second, SSA sought to act very promptly. Not only did the SSA interim criteria presume that simple CWP was compensable, it also resulted in compensation for other pulmonary or respiratory diseases, such as emphysema and bronchitis, as well. What were critical were the values considered as normal or below normal for the ventilatory tests. By setting a high standard on the "normal" level, the door was opened through these test standards for many previously denied claimants as well as for new ones.

There are several ways to gauge the ventilatory test standards that were set for claimants or survivors. First, a comparison between the permanent criteria and the interim criteria can readily be made since both appeared in the same issue of the *Federal Register.* It is clear that the values in the interim presumptions are set much higher than in the permanent standards. The higher the threshold is set, the larger the number of applicants that fall below it, enlarging the set of compensable applicants.

Second, at the time of the hearings on the 1977 amendments, numerous physicians commented on the interim presumptions. The consensus of their testimony was that, because the threshold was set so high, the standards were far too low. In addition, the standards were technically flawed by not being age-adjusted. Since ventilatory capacity typically declines with age, a "normal" value for a 65-year-old will be lower than for a 45-year-old. By not adjusting for age, the interim presumptions provided a boost for those claimants who were older, which is to say, the large bulk of the claimant population.

Aside from the age adjustment issue, a "normal" figure does not necessarily imply that everyone falling below that level is sick. With normal variation in the populations, persons without impairment often have capacities below the average, their age aside, so that impairment is not demonstrated simply because one's ventilatory tests place them below the "normal" figure. If the test takes age into account and perhaps certain other measurable factors, and the person's ventilatory capacity is perhaps 60 percent of the normal figure or less, one can then presume the presence of a significant impairment. This was what the medical community told the Perkins committee in 1977.[43]

Dr. Harold I. Passes, former acting Chief Medical Officer of the Bureau of Hearing and Appeals for SSA testified on the development of the interim standards during hearings on the 1977 amendments.[44] According to him, the interim standards were never given official medical approval by the Chief Medical Officer of the Bureau of Disability Insurance for SSA. Instead, "The criteria were designed for expediency by the then Bureau director, Mr. Popick, a nonphysician, and drafted by Mr. O'Brien, the chief legal counsel at the time."[45] Thereafter, lay personnel used the criteria 99.9 percent of the time without seeking medical advice. The interim criteria were

> . . . extremely liberal and were not based on substantial medical evidence that the criteria chosen were in fact, equal to a disabling impair-

ment. They did include many values, including pulmonary function standards, which were entirely normal and which would be read by at least 95 percent of all physicians who were knowledgeable of the values presented as normal values.[46]

Bernard Popick, who ran the Part B program in SSA, had been the focus for much of the criticism about the standards used by SSA until the 1972 amendments went into effect. The use of the interim criteria allowed him to respond to the heat directed at him and his office by black lung supporters, particularly in the Congress. The weight of the medical testimony regarding these criteria was that they were so liberal as to provide benefits to many claimants who suffered little or no impairment. As Solomons concludes, "The interim presumption began life a sort of dark secret, contrived by federal agency personnel who probably saw their careers flash before their eyes as a few powerful members of Congress grew more and more strident in their demands that more claims be paid."[47]

The interim criteria applied by SSA beginning in 1973 created a special problem for the Department of Labor. When their time came to administer claims under Part C, they were required to use the "permanent criteria" which were more demanding than the interim criteria. This created the almost laughable situation of two federal agencies administering essentially the same program, using substantially different standards to determine compensability. The circumstance was hardly considered laughable at the Labor Department, however, where the denial rate on claims was much higher than at the Social Security Administration. The criticism that had been heaped on SSA by black lung supporters before the enactment of the 1972 amendments soon was redirected at the Labor Department with its more restrictive standards. The Department's frustration was easy to understand. Since the statute appeared to give standard-setting power only to the Secretary of Health, Education and Welfare, the Labor Department felt trapped by the permanent standards it was required to employ. (In particular, this was dictated by sections 402(f) and 411.) In its first 18 months of administering the program, the Labor Department's approval rate was below 20 percent while SSA's approval rate had risen to over 60 percent, using their interim criteria.

Some evidence of the Labor Department's desperation can be inferred from their report on the program submitted in 1976 to Congress.[48] Apparently to explain the large number (and proportion) of claims denials, the Department reported on a sampling of 1,388 denials where ventilatory test results were available.[49] Of these, only 78 (6 percent) met the Labor Department's standard for benefit eligibility (and therefore had been denied on some other grounds), while 318 (23 percent) met the interim standards but not those of the Labor Department. This demonstrates tangibly the consequence of the use of the interim presumptions by SSA and the reason for the far lower acceptance rate by the Labor Department.

In 1975, SSA apparently agreed, at the Labor Department's urging, to extend the interim presumptions to the Part C program, but the effort was quietly killed by the Office of Management and Budget, according to Solomons.[50] Until then, the Labor Department's wish to use these more liberal standards was not based on any medical or scientific study. Instead, it was simply a desire to have the two agencies use the same standards, to take the heat off the Labor Department.

In March 1976, the House passed HR 10760, in which it provided that no claims were to be evaluated on the basis of criteria that were more strict than those applied by SSA in the interim presumptions. This bill would have permitted the

Department of Labor to use even more liberal criteria than the interim presumptions, but the issue became moot as the Senate was unable to complete work on the bill before the legislative session ended.

By the time the 95th Congress began work on a black lung reform bill, a Democratic administration was in place at the Labor Department, and a new perception of the interim presumptions surfaced there. According to Solomons,

> What happened, in fact, was that the Social Security Administration finally made it clear to Department of Labor officials that the interim presumption was scientifically invalid and that it was used by them, not as a screening device to separate appropriate claims from potential denials, but as an irrebuttable presumption which would permit the approval of large numbers of marginal claims with a minimum of effort and without full adjudication.[51]

The result of this remarkable shift by the Labor Department placed the new administration at odds on this critical issue with the powerful congressional advocates of liberalized standards. The Department adopted the position that medical knowledge should be employed to develop justifiable medical criteria. Indeed, the Senate's version of the Black Lung Benefits Reform Act of 1977 (BLBRA-1977) empowered the Secretary of Labor in consultation with the National Institute of Occupational Safety and Health to issue medical criteria. The House version, on the other hand, required the Labor Department to apply the interim presumptions to all its claims, including those previously denied.

A compromise of sorts was accepted by the Conference Committee whereby standards no more restrictive than the interim presumptions were to be applied, but only until the Labor Department adopted new permanent medical criteria.[52] At that point, evaluation of all subsequent claims would be based on the new standards. Very shortly after the amendments became effective, the Department proposed "interim" regulations of its own to interest groups and congressional staffers. Solomons reports that parts of the draft version were "severely criticized" and that the Department was compelled to back off most of the ones that appeared to tighten regulations.[53] The Department clearly complied with the legislative mandate that required these interim regulations to be no stricter than the interim presumptions used by SSA. Ultimately, the interim regulations proposed on April 25, 1978 were consistent with the Department's need to close out the enormous backlog of cases that had accumulated, along with the reevaluation of previously denied claims required under BLBRA-1977.

A final version of the permanent regulations was issued in February 1980, to be effective one month hence. The permanent standards were more rigorous than the interim standards had been. Thus, from the effective date of the amendments, March 1, 1978, the Labor Department had two years in which to administer the law using the SSA interim standards—and in so doing, to reduce the mountainous load of backed-up claims.

One way of assessing the significance of the Labor Department's use of the interim standards is available. The General Accounting Office studied 450 claim files taken as a random sample in 1980.[54] Almost all of these claims had been evaluated on the basis of the interim standards. GAO found that 205 claims had been approved from this sample, but that only 111 of these claims would have been accepted had the permanent standards been used instead. If the interim criteria had not been available, fully 45 percent of the accepted claims would have been denied. While this heftier denial rate would likely have reduced the volume of new claims, it would also have left the department with an enormous backlog of appeals and unresolved claims, to say nothing of the wrath of the black lung supporters in the Congress.

Disability

To this point, the focus of this chapter has been on the nature of the disease compensated under the black lung program and the methods used to determine whether the disease is present. Closely related issues created a variety of other serious problems for program administrators and for all parties involved with the system. These issues related to the requirement that living claimants be totally disabled as a condition of benefit eligibility. The concept of total disability is not as straightforward as Congress may have supposed it to be in 1969. To see why, some reference to other programs is necessary.

To help clarify what is meant by the term "disability," it is useful to distinguish it from the term "impairment." Impairment is strictly a medical or physiological (or psychological) concept, referring to the outcome of an injury, disease or possibly a genetic disorder. The extent of the impairment is a measure of the loss or disorder in purely medical or scientific terms. An impairment may be life threatening or relatively trivial in terms of limiting an individual's physical or psychological abilities.

Disability, by contrast, refers to the social and/or economic loss resulting from an impairment. Thus, in most compensation and liability systems, the major component of disability is the loss of income due to a partial or total loss of work-related income. If a compensation system is based totally on impairment, two persons suffering precisely the same anatomical loss would receive equal benefits. The loss of a single finger would be valued the same for a concert pianist as it would be for a real estate salesperson. By contrast, a pure disability system would provide equal benefits to workers with precisely the same economic losses, even if their impairments are vastly different. The loss of a finger for a professional pianist could conceivably be considered totally disabling, and comparable to the loss of both legs or both eyes for a laborer. Indeed, compensation might be greater for the pianist if that person's income loss was greater than that of the laborer.

Workers' compensation systems were originally conceived of as disability- and not impairment-based.[55] As such, the movement by a number of states in recent years toward a purer "wage loss approach" should perhaps be considered less a revolution than a return to the basics. In any case, there are numerous elements in workers' compensation systems within the U.S. and abroad that compromise the strict "disability principle," with added elements of an "impairment approach."

Just as workers' compensation systems are impure disability schemes, so too is the Social Security Disability Insurance (SSDI) program. In broad terms, the disability elements of SSDI are found in at least three features of the scheme. First, benefits are paid only where there has been a loss of earnings. Second, benefit levels are related to the applicant's previous level of earnings. Third, SSDI benefits are terminated when the recipient achieves retirement age (and retirement benefits are paid thereafter). The source of the disability, however, must be a "severe" impairment. Thus, SSDI deviates from a strict disability approach, since benefits would not be provided where a "non-severe" impairment results in a serious disability (loss of earnings).

This very cursory review of these concepts should clarify at least one other difference between impairment and disability. Medical and health specialists are better equipped than anyone to evaluate the extent of impairment. Disability, however, is best judged by nonmedical people, such as vocational and labor market experts, economists, or others trained to assess the degree of economic loss. Since many compensation jurisdictions leave the assessment of "disability" to physicians, it is little wonder that confusion has arisen over the basis for compensation benefits, much less over the terminology.

A critical distinction in compensation systems exists between those that provide benefits for partial disability, and those that do not. Partial disability benefit programs are complicated and difficult to administer. All of the states administer such programs under their workers' compensation laws, as does the federal government under the Federal Employees' Compensation Act. One of the inherent challenges of a partial disability system turns out to be a source of a certain strength. Where compensation or benefits are available only for total disability, there is little or no room for compromise or for legitimate uncertainty. For example, under the SSDI system with its all or nothing approach, decisions that are "wrong" are totally wrong. In a total disability-only program, benefits are paid to a person with 100 percent disability, but not to a person judged to be only 95 percent disabled (or some other appropriate threshold point). By contrast, compensation for partial disability allows the administering agency some room for movement, whether this be done to achieve compromise or to deal with uncertainties. "Errors" in judgment by the agency need not be of an "all or nothing" character.

All of this serves as background to the black lung program, which, in theory at least, compensated living applicants solely for totally disabling pneumoconiosis. Had the program been designed instead to compensate for partial disability, many of the program's difficulties would have been eliminated, though other problems undoubtedly would have surfaced. The question arises why Congress did not design a partial disability program. The record provides little to answer this question. One of the major supporters of the legislation in 1969, 1972 and 1977 was Congressman John H. Dent (D-Pennsylvania) who explained:

> The reason we rejected the partial basis was because we knew that they (Great Britain) paid it on a partial basis because they did not want to pay it on a final basis. They pay you so much—a couple of dollars more a week if you are in the first stage, and a couple of dollars more a week if you are in the second stage. In other words, they want to keep you in the mines so they decided to pay partial benefits. It is wrong and that is why it is wrong in Pennsylvania and it would be wrong here to do so.[56]

Dent's argument can be attacked on several grounds, the most obvious of which is that a partially disabled miner would more likely be able to leave the mines if he received a partial benefit than if he received none at all. Moreover, the level of total disability benefits under black lung was low enough to keep mine work relatively attractive, even to seriously impaired miners.[57]

It seems likely that Congress did not want to tackle the difficult chore of creating a partial disability program for a program that was to revert over (or back) to the states in a few years. Also, the language in the original Senate and House bills that went to the Conference Committee in 1969 dealt with complicated pneumoconiosis. Since a widely held view was that this condition was usually totally disabling, there was no need to provide for a partial disability system.

The distinction between impairment and disability highlights one of the special difficulties encountered in the program. Total disability implies a complete loss of earnings or earnings capacity due to injury or disease. Consequently, persons who have not worked because of advanced age, and who suffer no earnings loss when disease develops, can hardly be considered totally disabled, though they may suffer significant impairment.

The entire issue of work, retirement and disability takes on a special character when applied to coal mining. As noted in chapter 1, the huge loss of jobs in that sector in the 1950s and 1960s created many retirements that were essentially premature and involuntary. The location of the mining regions, especially those in the East where employment declines were greatest, were in regions that provided few alternative sources of employment. Generally, displaced miners found few opportunities, either in the mining areas or elsewhere. For these miners, loss of earnings was linked more to the economics of coal than to the result of an impairment. Additionally, miners with obvious impairments were handicapped in competing for any vacant positions that might open in the mines. To what extent was the loss of income suffered by these miners a result of economic circumstances and to what extent was it a result of the impaired condition?

The original law of 1969 dealt with the issue simplistically. Section 402(f) stated: "The term 'total disability' has the meaning given it by regulations of the Secretary of Health, Education and Welfare, but such regulations shall not provide more restrictive criteria than those applicable under section 223(d) of the Social Security Act." That section referred to the SSDI program, with which SSA had considerable experience.

The interpretation of the Conference Committee's thinking differed in each chamber. The analysis in the Senate stated, "The parameters of the term 'total disability' will be established from time-to-time by the Secretary of Health, Education and Welfare, but he must not establish more restrictive criteria for determining disability than the criteria applicable under section 223(d) of the Social Security Act, as amended, for purposes of disability under that Act. It is expected that initially this criteria [sic] will be followed. As time goes on, the Secretary may develop more liberal criteria consistent with the purpose of this title."[58]

In the House of Representatives, the analysis made no mention of eventual liberalization of the criteria. It did state, however: "Such standards would, among other things, require that the administrators of this program apply the best medical means available for ascertaining the disease in the miner."[59] It seems clear from this statement that the House, in particular, and likely the Senate as well, confused questions of diagnosis with those of disability. A working miner, for example, could be diagnosed as impaired with CWP, but would not be considered disabled under SSDI because of his employment status. A 65-year-old retired miner would normally not be eligible for SSDI, because of his age. By making the black lung benefit one based on impairment, it created a new sort of entity for SSA to administer. The agency was to apply the impairment criteria of section 223(d), but not necessarily the disability tests which were based on any loss of earnings and being below retirement age.

At least one issue involving disability was made perfectly clear, although its medical basis might have been shaky. Where a (former) miner was diagnosed as having complicated pneumoconiosis, section 411(c) (3) created an irrebuttable presumption that he was totally disabled due to pneumoconiosis. In this case, continued work in coal mining could not be used to deny benefits since the presumption was irrebuttable.

Where the miner was found to have some impairment from pneumoconiosis, benefits could be paid if that condition prevented the worker ". . . from doing coal mining work and from engaging in any other type of substantial gainful activity consistent with his vocational competence."[60] This left open the issue that SSA normally did not face under SSDI, that is, what to do with the 65-year-old applicant who was no longer employed. Essentially, what SSA did was to waive, effectively, any work test and base benefits solely on impairment criteria. For older miners short of retirement age, the work test was applied liberally: ". . . the older, long-term miner with minimal education and skills, who is shown to be unable to do heavy work because of pneumoconiosis, will ordinarily be found to be totally disabled."[61]

SSA's handling of the total disability question proved to be unsatisfactory and unacceptable to the supporters of the program and led to a change in the definition of total disability in the 1972 amendments. Under SSDI, a continuation of work by an applicant demonstrated the absence of total disability. Further, if an applicant's impairment was judged to be no deterrent to the person's taking gainful employment, SSDI benefits would be denied also. In applying these familiar concepts and regulations, seemingly consistent with the legislative requirement that the agency be no more restrictive in evaluating total disability than under SSDI, SSA earned the enmity of the congressional supporters of the program.

> The Committee believes that experience in the administration of the black lung benefit provisions to date reflects the need to modify the definition of disability applied in the adjudication of claims

under these provisions. The Committee makes no judgment on whether the test in title II of the Social Security Act 'inability to engage in any substantial gainful activity,' is an appropriate definition of application to the total universe of workers in the nation. But, it is unrealistic when applied to coal miners, if it results in the denial of claims of miners who for medical reasons can no longer be expected to work in the mines and for whom there is, too often, no other realistic employment opportunity, or for whom the only opportunity for employment may be at wages far less than they would have earned had they been able to continue to work in their usual jobs.[62]

The Committee's report went on to provide a much broader definition of total disability and to snipe at SSA for disregarding the intent expressed by Congress in 1969. Ultimately, something short of the Committee's proposed redefinition was passed, but it substantially widened the scope from that applied by SSA until 1972. This new version defined total disability in a miner as "when pneumoconiosis prevents him from engaging in gainful employment requiring the skills and ability comparable to those of any employment in a mine or mines in which he previously engaged with some regularity and over a substantial period of time."[63]

This revised definition carried in the 1972 amendments meant that working miners (even aside from those with complicated pneumoconiosis and covered by the irrebuttable presumption) could be considered totally disabled. So long as the miner's work no longer was in his usual line of coal mining employment, his working could not be used as grounds for denying the claim due to a finding of no total disability. It is necessary to note, however, that the awarding of benefits did not necessarily mean that payments would be made to working miners. Under the Part B program, SSA was able to offset, partially at least, black lung benefits paid where miners continued to have earnings. However, no such offset existed in the Part C program, so that total disability benefits could be paid to working miners. This practice was eliminated by the insertion of an offset provision under Part C in the 1981 amendments.[64]

The 1977 amendments reflect the realization by Congress that it had not satisfactorily solved the total disability issue in 1972. A number of matters arose that persuaded Congress that it had not gone far enough in 1972. First, some working miners were denied benefits for total disability due to pneumoconiosis because they continued to work in their long-term employment. Their continuing employment reflected the need they had for some source of income, combined with the long delays in processing and adjudicating claims in the Labor Department. Black lung supporters argued that the impaired miner was "carried" by fellow miners who assisted the person in doing his work. To deny benefits for total disability simply because the worker was still working at his long-term employment seemed unfair to them, and smacked of a Catch-22. Consequently, one of the changes in the rather lengthy definition provided by the 1977 amendments provided that, if a miner's employment conditions were changed, indicating the miner's reduced ability to do his usual coal mine work, such employment could not be used as conclusive evidence that the miner was not totally disabled. This meant that a working miner could file a claim and receive a positive benefit determination while still employed in a coal mine. However, in order to receive benefits, the miner would have to terminate that employment within one year after the eligibility determination had been made. (From section 413(d).)

A second matter dealt with by the 1977 amendments was the treatment by program administrators of certain survivors' claims. A number of complaints had reached congressional supporters of the program, that survivors' claims were being denied where the miner still had been employed in coal mining at the time of death. Presumably, such evidence was interpreted by the Department of Labor to mean that the miner was not totally disabled due to pneumoconiosis at the time of death. Such an interpretation seriously jeopardized the survivors' chances of obtaining benefits.

The argument for liberalizing the treatment of such claims was based on two factors. First, as we have just seen, Congress was prepared to accept the argument that a miner might be totally disabled but still employed in coal mining. If it insisted on this for living miner claimants, consistency compelled Congress to accept that some deceased miners who worked in the mines until they died also might have been totally disabled. Second, had that miner succeeded in obtaining black lung benefits while still alive, his survivors would have been entitled to benefits, regardless of the cause of his death (section 412(a) (2)). The result of this line of argument was that Congress pushed ahead in 1977 with, ". . . a deceased miner's employment in a mine at the time of death shall not be used as conclusive evidence that the miner was not totally disabled. . . ."[65] By making this decision, Congress greatly enhanced the chances for success by claimants wishing to invoke either the 15-year presumption (section 411(c) (4)), or the 25-year presumption (section 411(c) (5)).[66] The latter presumption, added in 1977, was the only place in the law, as amended, that ever made any reference to partial disability. It provided that for certain survivors' claims, benefits were to be paid if the miner, at the time of death, was either partially or totally disabled due to pneumoconiosis. Partial disability was not defined in the statute.

Under SSDI, benefits for total disability are frequently cut off when the recipient's condition improves, either medically or in terms of the labor market. SSA and the Labor Department, accustomed to that approach, did not treat benefits to living miners as automatic lifetime awards. When some recipients returned to work, for example, or when some incident occurred to suggest that the miner's impairment was not severe enough to cause total disability, the miner might be subject to reexamination.

While very few recipients actually had their benefits terminated, the possibility that this could occur upset black lung supporters. In response to regulations proposed by the Labor Department that had appeared earlier in the *Federal Register,* Congressmen Perkins, Simon and Dent wrote the Labor Department:

> We believe that the new rule in Part 718 relating to the reexamination of beneficiaries for the purpose of reaffirming a miner's continued eligibility for benefits represents a dangerous threat to the mental and physical well-being of the beneficiaries, and can easily be construed as an ill-conceived and miscast attempt by the Department of Labor to strip deserving individuals of their hard-won rights to benefits.[67]

This pressure, along with the statement that "the overwhelming majority of comments on this section suggest that it be stricken,"[68] forced the Labor Department to back off. Once benefits were awarded the miner could expect them to continue for life.

The problem with reexamination, as with most of the troublesome issues, was that the agencies continued to harbor notions of disability, while Congress was more intent on paying for impairment. By making such a choice, Congress allowed currently employed persons, even some still employed in the mines, to successfully pursue claims. More significantly, the impairment approach opened the door for thousands of older, nonworking, former miners to file claims and receive benefits. That characteristic of the program is clearly reflected in the available data on the ages of applicants and beneficiaries. For the first two full years of the program, 77 percent of living applicants under the Part B program were 60 years or older, and over 60 percent were 65 years or older.[69] Almost 73 percent of the allowed claims came from persons aged 65 years and older. Indeed, 70 percent of the miner beneficiaries were also collecting retirement benefits under Social Security.

The Labor Department's experience under Part C also reflects the tendency for the program to benefit older applicants. For example, by the end of 1975, more than 83 percent of the successful applicants were 61 years of age or older at the time of filing, and 46 percent of the living beneficiaries were 70 years or older at the time they filed.[70] The average age of miner beneficiaries under Part C was 67.4 years as of December 1979.[71]

Once the Part C program brought mine operators into the picture, they challenged the notion that total disability could exist where the claimant was still employed. Ultimately, the matter was dealt with by the U.S. Supreme Court, which appeared to identify the core issue: ". . . destruction of earning capacity is not the sole legitimate basis for compulsory compensation of employees. We cannot say that it would be irrational for Congress to conclude that impairment of health alone warrants compensation."[72]

The Supreme Court's decision addressed the issue of the authority of Congress to associate some degree of impairment with total disability. The Court found that Congress had acted within its powers, though it did not speak to the matter of the wisdom of doing so. Evidence of pneumoconiosis, even of the complicated categories, does not by itself mean the employee is disabled. "The chest X-ray is not a useful means of assessing the functional status of the lung nor of determining disability."[3] Nevertheless, with many retired miners showing some evidence of impairment, the intent of Congress was absolutely clear, as exemplified by the 1972 amendments and by the 1977 changes that followed.

NOTES

1. A discussion of these issues as they pertain to occupational disease and workers' compensation outside of black lung is found in Peter S. Barth with H. Allan Hunt, *Workers' Compensation and Work-Related Illnesses and Diseases* (Cambridge: MIT Press, 1980), chapters 3 and 4.

2. Much of the following review is based on Howard Rockette, *Mortality Among Coal Miners Covered by the UMWA Health and Retirement Funds* (Morgantown, W. VA: NIOSH, 1977) and Attilio D. Renzetti, Jr., et al., *Current Medical Methods in Diagnosing Coal Workers' Pneumoconiosis,* and *A Review of the Medical and Legal Definitions of Related Impairment and Disability,* prepared for the U.S. Department of Labor, Employment Standards Administration, Franklin Research Center, May 13, 1983. Some of their work is taken from A. Meiklejohn, "History of Lung Diseases of Coal Miners in Great Britain," Part I, 1800-1875 and Part II, 1874-1920, *British Journal of Industrial Medicine* 8:127, 1951 and 9:93, 1952.

3. Rockette et al., *Mortality Among Coal Miners,* p. 1.

4. The President's Commission on Coal, *The American Coal Miner: A Report on Community and Living Conditions in the Coalfields,* Washington, D.C., 1980, p. 120.

5. An excellent summary for lay persons of characteristics of the disease, along with the medical nomenclature is found in N. LeRoy Lapp, "A Lawyer's Medical Guide to Black Lung Litigation," *West Virginia Law Review* 83, 4 (Summer 1981), pp. 721-762.

6. *Coal Workers' Pneumoconiosis—Medical Considerations, Some Social Implications,* Mineral Resources and the Environment, Supplementary Report, National Academy of Sciences, Washington, D.C., 1976, pp. 5-6.

7. See Draft Report, Conference on Major Issues Raised in Study of Current Medical Methods Used in Diagnosing Coalworkers' Pneumoconiosis—Summary of Discussions, April 2-3, 1984, Franklin Research Center, p. 20.

8. Submission to the U.S. Department of Labor, June 14, 1978.

9. This section is based on Lapp, "Lawyer's Guide."

10. See *Coal Workers' Pneumoconiosis,* p. 9.

11. Ibid., p. 46.

12. Ibid., p. 5.

13. See W. Keith Morgan, Hearing before the Subcommittee on Oversight of the Committee of Ways and Means, House of Representatives, July 27 and September 28, 1981. Much of the following is based on his testimony and that of Dr. J. Donald Millar, director of NIOSH, at the same hearing.

14. See NIOSH testimony, ibid., p. 33.

15. See Millar testimony, ibid.

16. See Morgan testimony, ibid., p. 235.

17. *Legislative History of the Federal Coal Mine Health and Safety Act of 1969,* Part 2, prepared for the Subcommittee on Labor, U.S. Senate, 1975, p. 1955.

18. Section 402(b).

19. See *Federal Register,* Vol. 43, No. 80, April 25, 1978, section 718.201.

20. Ibid., Vol. 45, No. 42, February 29, 1980.

21. Ibid., Vol. 43, No. 80, section 718.201.

22. See U.S. Steel Corporation v. Gray, 588 F. 2d. 1022 n.3 (5th Cir. 1979) cited in *Black Lung Desk Book,* Benefits Review Board, U.S. Department of Labor, August 1981, iv-14.

23. Specifically, the margin occurs at readings of 0/1 and 1/0.

24. Testimony submitted to U.S. Department of Labor, June 1978.

25. Testimony submitted by Dr. William Cole to the U.S. Department of Labor, June 14, 1978.

26. Testimony to the U.S. Department of Labor, June 1978.

27. Ibid.

28. Hearings before the Subcommittee on Oversight of the Committee of Ways and Means, U.S. House of Representatives, July 27, September 28, 1981, Serial 97-32, p. 39.

29. Testimony submitted to the U.S. Department of Labor, June 14, 1978.

30. *Black Lung Program Manual,* U.S. Department of Labor, February 1980, Chap. 2-501, p. 35.

31. *Black Lung Benefits Program,* First Annual Report (of SSA) on Part B of Title IV of the Federal Coal Mine Health and Safety Act of 1969, Committee on Education and Labor, House of Representatives, Committee Print, 1971, p. 18.

32. Ibid.

33. Ibid.

34. Ibid.

35. Second Annual Report to Congress on the Administration of Part B of Title IV of the Federal Coal Mine Health and Safety Act of 1969, SSA Pub. No. 80-72 (11-72), table 3.

36. Report No. 92-743, to accompany HR 9212, Senate, April 10, 1972, p. 18.

37. Ibid.

38. See Report No. 92-460, August 5, 1971.

39. Mark E. Solomons, "A Critical Analysis of the Legislative History Surrounding the Black Lung Interim Presumptions and a Survey of its Unresolved Issues," *West Virginia Law Review,* Vol. 83, Summer 1981, p. 878.

40. Paragraph 410.490, p. 20645.

41. Ibid. See also *Black Lung Benefits Program,* Third Annual Report of Part B of Title IV of the Federal Coal Mine Health and Safety Act of 1969, January 1974, printed for the Committee on Education and Labor, House of Representatives, p. 97.

42. Ibid.

43. Hearings before the Committee on Education and Labor, House of Representatives, 95th, 1st session, March 14-17, 21, 1977.

44. Ibid.

45. Ibid., p. 274.

46. Ibid., pp. 274-275.

47. Solomons, "Critical Analysis," p. 915.

48. *Black Lung Benefits Act of 1972,* Second Annual Report on Administration of the Act During Calendar Year 1975, U.S. Department of Labor, July 1976.

49. Ibid., p. 29.

50. Solomons, "Critical Analysis," p. 886.

51. Ibid., pp. 890-891.

52. Section 402(f).

53. Solomons, "Critical Analysis," p. 896.

54. Report to the Congress, Legislation Authorized Benefits without Adequate Evidence of Black Lung or Disability, GAO, January 19, 1982. The study is discussed more fully in chapter 6.

55. See C. Arthur Williams, Jr. and Peter S. Barth, *Compendium on Workmen's Compensation,* National Commission on State Workmen's Compensation Laws, Washington, D.C., 1973, Chap. 3.

56. Hearings before the Committee on Education and Labor, 95th Congress, 1st session, March 14-17, 21, 1977, p. 25.

57. Benefits are described in chapter 6.

58. *Legislative History,* Part 2, p. 1622.

59. *Legislative History,* Part 2, p. 1532.

60. See *Federal Register,* 20 CFR 410.403 b.

61. *Black Lung Benefits Program,* First Annual Report, p. 8.

62. Report No. 92-743 from the Committee on Labor and Public Welfare, U.S. Senate, to accompany Black Lung Benefits Act of 1972, HR 9212, April 12, 1972, pp. 16-17.

63. Section 402(f).

64. See the discussion on offsets in chapter 6 and on the 1981 amendments in chapter 7.

65. Section 402(f) (1) (B) (i).

66. Presumptions are discussed in chapter 4.

67. Correspondence addressed to Robert Dorsey, July 11, 1978.

68. See the proposed regulations in the *Federal Register,* section 718.404, April 28, 1978, and the final regulations in the *Federal Register,* February 19, 1980.

69. See table 4, *Black Lung Benefits Program,* Second Annual Report.

70. *Black Lung Benefits Act of 1972:* Second Annual Report, pp. 25-27.

71. *Black Lung Benefits Act:* Annual Report on Administration of the Act during Calendar Year 1979, p. 35.

72. Usery v. Turner-Elkhorn Mining Co., 96 S. Ct. 2896, 428 U.S. 23 (1976).

73. *Coal Workers' Pneumoconiosis.*

• 4 •
Presumptions and Evidence

Workers or survivors seeking state workers' compensation benefits for disability or death due to occupational diseases typically encounter significant difficulties.[1] There is no need to dwell here on the results of this pattern. Suffice it to point to the difficulties for compensation purposes posed by diseases of long latency or of unknown etiology, or by diagnostic uncertainties, exposures to multiple hazards both on the job and away from it, limited information regarding the extent of the hazardous exposure, and so on. The special difficulty that the worker or survivor must contend with is that, with very rare exceptions, the claimant must shoulder the burden of proof. Providing the proof necessary to win benefits in state proceedings can be extremely difficult, if not impossible. Some workers' compensation laws seek to reduce or to shift some of that burden away from claimants in order to increase the likelihood of their winning benefits. The purpose of this chapter is to examine the manner in which the legislation dealt with these issues of providing proof and adequate evidence for black lung claimants.

Presumptions

The 1969 legislation and the amendments in 1972 and 1977 sought to provide benefits to miners or to survivors where coal mine employment was responsible for death or disability due to pneumoconiosis. Beginning in 1969, and with the

109

next two sets of amendments, Congress attempted to ease the customary burden of proof on claimants, thereby increasing the probability of benefits being awarded. What all claimants needed to prove, minimally, was that:

- the disease arose out of coal mine employment;
- the disease was pneumoconiosis;
- the disease was totally disabling or was the cause of death.

In 1969, and even more so subsequently, supporters of the law understood at least some of the challenges to claimants posed by the need to prove these matters. The whole matter of how to diagnose the presence of pneumoconiosis was wide open in 1969. Compounding this, facilities to provide sophisticated examinations to miners were inadequate at that time. Moreover, with the decision by the Congress to compensate old cases, how would the law cope with deaths that occurred in earlier years, particularly where no autopsy had been performed? The probative value of death certificates was recognized as being extremely limited. Finally, what would it take for the miner or his survivor to prove that the disease was caused by coal mining employment?

To deal with these issues and to ease, if not remove, the burden on the claimant to prove one or more of these difficult matters, Congress provided a number of presumptions in the original law. It is important to note that a presumption does not assure a claimant of being compensated. First, the presumption may involve only a single element of a claim, and where it is employed, the claimant must invariably prove other points as well in order to be compensated. (Some of those other matters to be proven can involve different presumptions.) Second, since most of the presumptions in this law simply shifted the burden of proof to the other party, i.e., the employer or the government, they could be rebutted. As such, the claimant might lose even on a matter where the presumption was invoked.

In another section, the issues of claimant eligibility are described. For purposes of understanding the presumptions in the law, it is sufficient to note that three sets of entitlements exist under the law. The original law provided that benefits were to be paid, "in respect of total disability of any miner due to pneumoconiosis and in respect of the death of any miner whose death was due to pneumoconiosis." (Section 411(a).) Thus, benefits were paid where there was an appropriately disabled living miner or where a claimant showed that a miner's death was caused by the disease. In the 1972 amendments, a third source of entitlement was added involving any deceased miner "who at the time of his death was totally disabled due to pneumoconiosis." This addition meant that a widow could receive benefits even where the miner had not made a claim for black lung by the time of his death and whose death could not have been caused by the disease, e.g., he died in an auto accident.[2] Moreover, this new entitlement meant that where a living miner had successfully pursued a black lung claim, his dependent survivors were assured of benefits upon his death, regardless of the cause of death.

Until the 1981 changes in law, there were seven presumptions that had been employed to aid the claimant in receiving benefits. Three of these are found in the 1969 law (sections 411(c) (1), (2) and (3)); a fourth was added in 1972 (411(c) (4)) and a fifth was added with the 1977 amendments (411(c) (5)). A sixth presumption was added by the Secretary of Labor's administrative regulations of 1978. Finally, Congress imposed a set of "interim presumptions" to be used in the 1977 amendments. Each is examined below. They are significant in several respects, the most important perhaps being that they reflect the attitude of the Congress towards the matter of compensating miners and their dependents.

Sections 411(c) (1) and (2) of the original law are broadly similar, though they have two significant differences. In

411(c) (1), the law establishes that "if a miner who is suffering or suffered from pneumoconiosis was employed for ten years or more in one or more coal mines there shall be a rebuttable presumption that his pneumoconiosis arose out of such employment."

Note that in order to invoke the presumption, the miner must have had ten or more years of coal mine employment. (With the 1972 amendments these years could have been spent in surface as well as underground mining.) This presumption, by itself, still left the claimant with the burden of proving that he did have pneumoconiosis. As long as the ten-year period of coal mine employment was shown, the presumption was invoked, essentially making the miner's other employment history irrelevant as a defense against the claim. Successful rebuttal of the presumption is difficult and rare in practice.

The Labor Department specifically identifies four lines of argument that are *not* sufficient to rebut the 411(c) (1) presumption:[3]

1. The presence of other lung conditions.
2. The presence of respiratory-pulmonary impairment prior to coal mine employment.
3. Additional dust exposure in other employment, either prior to or subsequent to the miner's coal mine employment.
4. Evidence that the mines where the miner worked were relatively dust-free.

Section 411(c) (2) provides that "if a deceased miner was employed for ten years or more in one or more coal mines and died from a respirable disease there shall be a rebuttable presumption that his death was due to pnneumoconiosis." This section differs from 411(c) (1) in several respects. First, it is meant to be invoked only in death claims. Second, its focus is on the cause of death and not on whether it arose out of coal mine employment. To invoke the presumption, the claimant must show only that the miner's death was due to a respirable disease, e.g., emphysema, etc. Having shown that, the presumption is that the disease was pneumoconiosis.

If the claimant can use this presumption, and it is not successfully rebutted, the claimant must also prove that the presumed pneumoconiosis arose out of coal mining employment. This is particularly simple since the ten or more years of coal mine employment that permit the use of 411(c) (2) can then be used to invoke 411(c) (1), allowing the claimant to presume also that the disease arose out of this employment.

It is difficult to rebut the section 411(c) (2) presumption. To do so requires that the government or the employer prove either of two rather difficult things. The rebuttal can be that the disease does not suggest a reasonable possibility that death was due to pneumoconiosis. The other available rebuttal is to prove that the respirable disease made a minimal or insignificant contribution to the miner's death. Where death is due to multiple causes including a respirable disease, and it is not medically feasible to distinguish which disease caused the death, death shall be found due to respiratory disease. At one point the Labor Department tentatively proposed excluding lung cancer and diseases of bacteriological or viral origin from diseases covered by the section 411(c) (2) presumption.[4] The proposal was not contained in the final regulations "since it is possible that a relationship between these diseases and exposure to coal mine dust and death may be established by medical evidence in a particular case."[5]

The Labor Department has interpreted section 411(c) (2) to apply to chronic respiratory diseases only. It was found that lung cancer is not chronic and, hence, the presumption has not been invoked where no other disease is present.

However, where the worker is found to have had pneumoconiosis or another chronic respiratory illness in addition to the lung cancer, the claimant may be able to employ this presumption. It seems clear that the Labor Department has had consistent difficulties in dealing with lung cancer cases in disabled or deceased miners.

For the claimant with less than ten years of coal mine employment, neither 411(c) (1) nor 411(c) (2) serve as negative presumptions, i.e., it is not to be presumed that the pneumoconiosis did *not* arise out of coal mine employment, nor that the respirable disease that killed the worker was not pneumoconiosis. The inability to invoke these (and the other) presumptions simply means that the claimant shoulders the burden of proof.

The third of the presumptions enacted in 1969 is unlike any of the other presumptions described here. Section 411(c) (3) states that where the miner suffers or suffered from complicated pneumoconiosis, there is an *irrebuttable* presumption that the miner is totally disabled due to pneumoconiosis, that his death was due to pneumoconiosis, or that at the time of death he was totally disabled by pneumoconiosis (added in 1972). The claimant still has the burden of proof that the disease arose out of the coal mine employment. However, where the miner was in coal mine employment for ten or more years, the section 411(c) (1) presumption can be invoked to meet this test.

The presence of complicated pneumoconiosis must be established as a fact by the administrative law judge.[6] Section 411(c) (3) provides some very limited guidance in defining three methods of establishing its presence, including the size of the opacities found in the miner's chest X-rays. Even where the miner remained employed in his usual coal mining job for four years after his X-ray revealed the existence of complicated pneumoconiosis, he was found totally disabled due to pneumoconiosis for this entire period because of section 411(c) (3).[7] The Supreme Court has upheld the use of this irrebuttable presumption in *Usery v. Turner-Elkhorn Mining Co.*[8]

The prevailing attitude in the Congress between 1970 and 1972 was one of considerable unhappiness among the program's advocates regarding the difficulty that miners and their survivors were encountering in obtaining benefits. Evidence accumulated by SSA as well as grass roots rumblings persuaded the law's principal supporters from the mining states that entitlements were too difficult to achieve under the existing administration of the act. As a result, the 1972 amendments created a new presumption, 411(c) (4), to make benefits available to more applicants.

The newer presumption is more complicated than those created in the original law. It states that where (1) a miner was employed for *15 years or more in undergound coal mines,* and (2) where a chest roentgenogram submitted in connection with the claim is interpreted as negative, and (3) where other evidence demonstrates the existence of totally disabling *respiratory or pulmonary impairment,* there shall be a presumption (rebuttable) that the miner is totally disabled to pneumoconiosis or that his death was due to pneumoconiosis. Where the claim involves a living miner, a wife's affidavit may not be used by itself to establish the presumption, according to the statute. The presumption, the subsection continues, may be used by miners employed in other than underground mines where the Labor Department finds that the employment conditions "were substantially similar to conditions in an underground mine." Unlike the earlier presumptions that appear in the law (411(c) (1) (2) and (3)), the 1972 addition specifies how the presumptions may be rebutted. To do so requires establishing that the miner does not or did not have pneumoconiosis or proving that the respiratory or pulmonary impairment did not arise out of or in connection with coal mine employment. The presumption was to be available only in old cases, where all 15 years or more of employment ended by July 1, 1971, and with certain limits on filing imposed by a statute of limitation. These time rules were dropped in the 1977 amendments and are therefore not considered here. July 1, 1971 was the date that certain, more restrictive dust standards went into effect under the coal Mine Health and Safety Act of 1969.

The newer presumption must be understood as being a significant extension of the intent of 411(c) (2), which applied only in death claims. It created an entitlement in living (former) miner claims for "presumptive pneumoconiosis." In death cases it went well beyond 411(c) (2) in widening eligibility since the earlier presumption required death due to a respiratory or pulmonary disease. Under 411(c) (4), the deceased miner with 15 years or more of coal mine employment could have died of any cause at all. For example, even if a miner died in an automobile accident, the presumption could be invoked to show that the miner was totally disabled from pneumoconiosis at the time of death, thereby creating an entitlement for his survivors.

For living claimants, this presumption cannot be used until it has been shown that the miner had a totally disabling, chronic respiratory or pulmonary disease. To do this, the living miner claimant must present some medical evidence of the existence of the disease, not solely lay testimony.[9] This requirement could be satisfied by the medical conclusion of at least one examining physician. In contrast to the living miner claim, lay evidence alone can establish that the miner was totally disabled due to pneumoconiosis at the time of death. Evidence such as a surviving spouse's affidavit is sufficient to trigger the presumption, where no other evidence exists or is brought forward to shed light on the claim. That the Congress intended this to be the case was clear. It was accomplished by explicitly providing that such an affidavit could not be used by itself to establish the presumption in living miner claims. The implications of this provision were that such an affidavit could be used in conjunction with other supportive evidence in living miner claims, and that it could be sufficient by itself where the miner was deceased. The rather minimal need for evidence to invoke 411(c) (4) in deceased miner claims became extremely controversial. Proponents argued, however, that survivors ought not to be denied benefits where the worker did have pneumoconiosis, but died at a time when there was little or no concern about establishing proper medical evidence.

The claimant must show, in order to use the presumption, that the miner is totally disabled, was totally disabled at the time of death, or died due to pneumoconiosis. Evidence that the miner died of a myocardial infarction and that he worked full-time without being "carried" by his co-workers until the mine closed prior to his death, would cause the Benefits Review Board to deny the survivor/claimant the use of the 411(c) (4) presumption.[10] The Board would find the miner not to have been totally disabled due to pneumoconiosis, nor to have died because of it.

As with 411(c) (2), there has been an inconsistent pattern of decisions involving lung cancer under 411(c) (4). In a recent decision, a survivor was permitted to invoke 411(c) (4) since lung cancer was a "totally disabling respiratory or pulmonary impairment."[11]

The two lines of argument that can be used to rebut 411(c) (4) are that the claimant does not or did not have pneumoconiosis, or that the impairment did not arise out of coal mine employment. Negative X-rays alone cannot be used as evidence of the absence of disease. Pulmonary function tests that do not meet the standards for total disability are not adequate to rebut the presumption. Negative X-rays *and* pulmonary function tests may be used to form a reasoned medical opinion that the disease is not present and, therefore, rebut the presumption.[12] An autopsy may also provide evidence of the absence of pneumoconiosis and permit the presumption to be rebutted. This leads to a considerable burden on the government or the employer to prove that there is no pneumoconiosis present.

Proving that the impairment did *not* arise out of coal mine employment can be difficult also. Even where a miner experienced a 30-year interval between his last coal mine employment and his initial effort to seek medical treatment for a lung condition, the employer was unable to rebut the presumption.[13] A number of cases exist where the employer failed to rebut on grounds that the impairment did not arise out of coal mine employment since there was no reasonable degree of medical certainty that the miner's emphysema was due to his cigarette smoking.[14]

The law allows surface miners to invoke 411(c) (4) where there is environmental comparability with an underground mine. The burden of proving comparable working conditions, which rests with the claimant, is discussed later in this section. However, an aboveground miner working at an underground mine is considered for these purposes to be an underground miner. Such a miner can use the presumption without having to show any appropriate dust exposure.

Following the 1972 amendments, black lung supporters in the Congress sought to extend entitlements even beyond the existing presumptions. They had recognized the enormous leverage that presumptions provided to claimants. Yet, they remained dissatisfied with the rate of claims approvals, so that they considered other presumptions to include in the law. Particularly attractive in this regard were presumptions that were made irrebuttable or, even more attractive, benefits based solely on the number of years employed in the mines. Numerous efforts were made to push through such broadened entitlements. In doing so, supporters of a more liberalized approach often gave up even the sheerest pretense that this was a disability or compensation scheme and, instead, in some instances manifested their preference for a straight pension scheme. A few examples of these are noted:

1. HR 8 was introduced by Congressman Dent and signed by Congressmen Perkins, Flood, et al. on January 14, 1975. Among other things, it provided that if a miner was employed for 25 years or more in underground mines, there was a rebuttable presumption that he was totally disabled, or at the time of his death was totally disabled, or his death was due to pneumoconiosis. Further, with 35 years or more in underground coal employment, there would be an irrebuttable presumption of total disability or death due to pneumoconiosis.

2. In February 1975, 17 congressmen introduced HR 2913, which would have created an irrebuttable presumption that a miner is totally disabled or has died due to pneumoconiosis after 15 years employment in underground coal mining. It would be applicable to surface miners who had worked in conditions substantially similar to underground miners.

3. HR 10760 was introduced much later in the first session of the same 94th Congress, November 14, 1975. Sponsored by Congressmen Dent, Flood, Perkins, Burton, et al., it provided that benefits be paid to miners or survivors after 30 years of underground employment; if the work was in anthracite mines, the period was shortened to 25 years. The familiar passage about substantially similar conditions would have brought many surface miners in under these proposed entitlements. The reasons for the position were spelled

out in the House Report that accompanied the bill from Perkin's Committee:

On June 23, 1973, pursuant to growing complaints regarding eligibility determination inequities, the Subcommittee conducted an oversight hearing in Eastern Kentucky, a major coal-producing area, and received testimony from more than 100 miners and widows who generally alleged wrongful denials of the benefit claims. Virtually all who appeared testified with regard to claims involving coal mining work exposures well in excess of 30 years. It was immediately apparent to the Subcommittee that the greatest number of the miner witnesses were severely and dramatically handicapped by respiratory difficulties. And it was equally apparent that the widows were testifying about the disabilities of husbands arising out of work experiences identical to those of the miners who appeared before the Subcommittee. Subsequent investigation revealed that the Eastern Kentucky universe was not unique in that respect; indeed, that many seemingly allowable claims involving miners with extended coal mining work experiences were curiously being denied. The justifications given in individual cases more often turned on disputed or unavailable medical evidence; and proved ultimately unsatisfactory to the Subcommittee, and thereafter to the full Committee as well.[15]

Having explained the source of their discontent, the Committee explained their proposed remedy:

In recognition of the historically demonstrated and exceedingly high probability of total disability (80.89 %), and out of concern for an equally probable risk of error in the remaining cases, an objective test was established to simply provide part B benefits payments to all claimants whose claims had been denied and who could demonstrate 30 or more years of underground coal mining experience. This assertedly rational and reasonable approach was elected over discretely restructuring the eligibility determination process in order to reach such legitimate and compelling cases: a restructuring, incidentally, which would have produced a complex, unmanageable, and enormously costly approach to ascertaining benefit entitlements.[16]

In short, the committee was expressing its anger with the executive branch's handling of black lung claims. (The 80.89 percent was the approval rate under Part B as of 1975.) Evidence that deserving miners and survivors were not being compensated was based on personal observation during the course of hearings held in Congressman Perkins' district. By limiting the presumption, at that point at least, to Part B claims, the higher program costs would have fallen on the U.S. Treasury, and not on the mine operators. Clearly, even 411(c) (4) had not gone far enough to suit the supporters of enlarged entitlements during this period.

Considerable resistance was encountered to adding any presumptions that would have conferred entitlement solely on the basis of years worked in coal mining. To have done this would have stripped away any semblance of a disability-based compensation program. The 1975 legislation (HR 10760) cleared the House by only 27 votes and no accommodation with the Senate could be worked out. Sensitive to this, Congressman Dent spoke on both sides of the issue in his testimony on the 1977 amendments:

Now I am hoping that we will not get into the question of carelessly saying only because of the number of years that this person worked in a mine, that person is totally disabled. We cannot simply write that as a principle of law. When we established the 30 years, we did it on the basis of very thorough research.[17]

The presumption that was added in the 1977 amendments was 411(c) (5). It dealt only with miners who had worked 25 or more years prior to June 30, 1971 (the date that stricter coal mine dust standards went into effect), and who died on or before March 1, 1978, the effective date of the new law. For such miners, the survivor claimant would receive benefits unless it could be proven that at the time of death the miner was not *partially* or totally disabled due to pneumoconiosis. It is notable that this is the only instance in the law's history where partial disability is compensable—though the level of benefits is no different from that awarded if death was due to pneumoconiosis.

The rationale for this presumption can be found in the *Legislative History:*

> Widows have perhaps been more adversely and wrongfully affected by black lung claim denials than living miners, for in all too many instances the probative value of the widow's evidence submitted in support of a claim is not good. It is not her fault. Medical records may have been lost or destroyed. The miner may have been lost forever in an underground mine explosion. He may have died so long ago that clinical knowledge of the day did not include pneumoconiosis—the cause of death was simplistically attributed to "heart failure." For these and other reasons the committee believes that concerns for the welfare of these widows, whose husbands gave their physical strength, their bodies and their lives to this most difficult occupation, should override any professed need to demonstrate

a clinically precise association between years worked and totally disabling lung disease.[18]

Since partial disability became an issue under 411(c) (5),
defining it became necessary. This was done in the Labor
Department's regulations. Partial disability was said to exist
where the miner had a reduced ability to engage in his usual
coal mine work or comparable and gainful work.[19]

In order to make use of this presumption, the survivor
needed only to show that the miner was employed for 25
years or more in coal mining—underground or otherwise—prior to June 30, 1971, and that the miner died on or
before March 1, 1978. The claimant was obliged to make
available any existing medical evidence, but did not need to
show that the miner was partially or totally disabled at the
time of death. Instead, it was the other party's burden to
prove that partial or total disability did not exist. Actually,
there are three possible rebuttals to the presumption:

1. The miner did not have pneumoconiosis.
2. The miner was not partially or totally disabled due to
   pneumoconiosis.
3. The miner's partial or total disability was not caused
   by pneumoconiosis.

The regulations spelled out four types of evidence that,
alone, would be insufficient to rebut the presumptions:[20]

1. Evidence that the deceased was employed in the mines
   at the time of his death.
2. Evidence pertaining to the deceased's level of earnings.
3. An X-ray that is negative.
4. A death certificate that contains no reference to
   pneumoconiosis.

However, the Benefits Review Board decided that two or
more of these may be sufficient to rebut the 25-year
presumption.[21]

The sixth presumption created under the law is essentially different from the ones noted above. Its focus is primarily on coverage under the act. It bears directly on 411(c) (1-5), however, as it may be used to determine whether or not these presumptions are applicable. The 1977 amendments considered a person who worked in coal mine construction or transportation as a miner "to the extent such individual was exposed to coal dust as a result of such employment."[22] It also differs from each of the presumptions described above since only this one was promulgated by regulation. The Secretary of Labor created a rebuttable presumption that "such individual was exposed to coal mine dust during all periods of such employment occurring in or around a coal mine or coal preparation facility. . . ."[23]

The presumption can be rebutted in two ways, according to the regulations. The employer or government must prove either that the miner was not regularly exposed to coal dust during the employment, or that the individual was not employed in or around a coal mine or preparation facility.

The final set of presumptions examined here is the so-called interim presumptions. The evolution of these standards for evaluating claims has already been described in this study. It is sufficient to observe here that they were developed by SSA in response to the 1972 amendments and the intense pressure from certain congressmen and senators to raise the approval rate under Part B claims. This result was accomplished through the implementation of the interim presumptions. The Labor Department sought to use these presumptions as well in administering Part C claims, but was prevented from doing so by the legality that prevented the Secretary of Labor from establishing the medical standards for purposes of determining the outcome of claims.

As an ultimate irony, by 1977 the Labor Department had become convinced that the interim presumptions that SSA continued to use were not medically sound, erring on the side of awarding benefits when that was unwarranted. However, the congressional mood in 1977 was to have the program further liberalized and, in particular, to raise the claims approval rate in the Labor Department. The House version of the bill would have imposed the application of the interim presumptions to all claims, forthcoming and previously filed but denied or pending that were to be reviewed again under the new criteria. The Senate version of the bill allowed the Secretary of Labor to draw up his own medical standards. The compromise that emerged from the Conference Committee imposed the application of criteria that were not more restrictive than the interim presumptions on the Labor Department for all reviewed claims (see Section 401(f) (2)), until that time that the Department promulgated a new set of standards. Claims filed until that time would be evaluated under the interim presumptions.

In August of 1978, the Labor Department published regulations implementing the criteria imposed on it by the 1977 law.[24] Basically, the presumptions are invoked where the miner had 10 or more years of coal mine employment and any one of five types of evidence are established:

1. A chest X-ray, biopsy or autopsy establishes the existence of pneumoconiosis.
2. Ventilatory studies establish the presence of a chronic respiratory or pulmonary disease.
3. Blood gas studies demonstrate impairment in the transfer of oxygen from the lung alveoli to the blood.
4. "Other medical evidence" establishes the presence of a totally disabling respiratory or pulmonary impairment. This can include the documented opinion of a physician using reasoned medical judgment.
5. Where the miner is deceased and where no other medical evidence is available, the affidavit of the sur-

vivor or other persons with knowledge of the condition can demonstrate the presence of a totally disabling pulmonary or respiratory impairment.

Where any of these five conditions is found alongside 10 or more years of coal mine employment, the miner "will be presumed to be totally disabled due to pneumoconiosis, or to have been totally disabled due to pneumoconiosis at the time of death, or death will be presumed to be due to pneumoconiosis, arising out of that employment. . . ."[25] This served to presume three critical elements for claimants: total disability, the presence of pneumoconiosis, and the disease having arisen out of coal mining employment. One of the keys to the presumptions was the ventilatory standards, which were set so high that many claimants would now be considered impaired and thereby able to invoke the presumptions. The use of "other medical evidence" and the widow's affidavit were also extremely important in aiding claimants.

There were four ways to rebut the interim presumptions:

1. Where the evidence establishes that the miner is doing his usual coal mine work or comparable and gainful work.
2. Where, in the light of all evidence, it is established that the individual is able to do his usual coal mine work or comparable and gainful work.
3. Where the evidence establishes that the total disability or death of the miner did not arise in whole or in part out of coal mine employment.
4. Where the evidence establishes that the miner does not or did not have pneumoconiosis.

Solomons discusses the controversy that developed within the Congress over the application of the interim presumptions by the Labor Department. He suggests that SSA had treated the presumptions *de facto* as irrebuttable, and that some, such as Senator Javits, insisted that this not be done by the Labor Department. Moreover, there was the related issue of whether the entire medical record should be considered by the administrative law judge in permitting the presumption to be invoked. The Department's position can be seen in Secretary Marshall's letter to President Carter, recommending that he sign the 1977 amendments:

> We are opposed to provisions making the use of the "interim standards" mandatory for the determination of total disability under Part C. . . . While we still believe the "interim standards" are inappropriate, the limitation of their use to reviewed and pending claims in conjunction with the requirement that all other relevant evidence be considered reduces our concerns substantially.[26]

The regulations that the Department issued subsequently were consistent with Marshall's concerns: "In adjudicating a claim under this subpart, all relevant medical evidence shall be considered."[27] The implication of this is that the interim presumptions were *administered* in a manner somewhat more restrictive than that of SSA. Nevertheless, the interim presumptions under either Parts B or C made many claimants' positions far simpler to sustain than had the pre-existing presumptions.

The publication of the Secretary of Labor's regulations on February 29, 1980 (effective date 3-31-80) meant that the interim presumptions could not be invoked in claims filed thereafter. In the 1981 amendments, the three other most controversial presumptions were dropped from the law: 411(c) (2) (10 years coal mine employment—death from respiratory-pulmonary cause presumed black lung); 411(c) (4) (15 years coal mine employment—presumptive pneumoconiosis if evidence of totally disabling respiratory-pulmonary disease); and 411(c) (5) (25 years coal mine employment—survivors presumption unless proven that partial or totally disabling pneumoconiosis not present).[28]

The presumptions under black lung are significant for several reasons. They provide a precise record of the extent to which Congress, SSA and the Labor Department sought to aid claimants. Second, the presumptions appear to have been the most pronounced feature of this federal program, at least among people involved with state workers' compensation systems. No other elements of the law seem to have deviated as much from existing practices under established state systems. Treated collectively, the presumptions under black lung have been widely viewed as the epitome of political manipulation of the pork barrel process, under the guise of operating a workers' compensation scheme.

Evidence

With hundreds of thousands of claims for benefits under the black lung program, SSA and the Department of Labor were forced to wrestle with numerous issues regarding the type and quality of evidence they would accept. It was one thing to set certain standards for determining whether a miner was disabled due to pneumoconiosis, but quite another to have the evidence to allow the determination to be made. If it was not clear in 1969, it became totally apparent by 1972, and certainly by 1977, that Congress did not wish to place major burdens of proof on the claimants. Consequently, the evidence required of claimants would be of a less demanding character than one could expect to find under typical state workers' compensation programs or in the SSDI program.

To highlight some of these issues, it is useful to separate claims that came from living miners from those of survivors. In the case of living miners, SSA basically followed the system that was familiar to it. Many claimants had had previous dealings with SSA, having applied for disability, retirement, or survivor benefits, and the agency had access to and used these data sources. SSA also sought and received access to state workers' compensation claims files, and it also used data from the Welfare and Retirement Fund of the United Mine Workers of America.[29] These steps permitted "a large number" of claims to be allowed with no need to obtain new evidence from applicants. Where miners did need to obtain medical examinations or reports, SSA either reimbursed applicants or paid the providers directly. Where the existing records were inadequate for SSA to make an assessment, the state agencies used for SSDI purposes were used also for black lung. These agencies arranged to have claimants examined by physicians and qualified facilities close to the claimants' residence. Unlike the situation in SSDI, this presented unusual problems for the agency because the claimants were so concentrated in a few areas, generally far removed from urban locations with their greater number of health care specialists and facilities. For example, over two-thirds of all pulmonary function tests scheduled for SSA applicants in the first 15 months of the program were in three states: Pennsylvania, West Virginia, and Kentucky.[30] The use of local providers was continued by the Labor Department when it took over the administration of the program.

In developing evidence to determine whether living claimants were totally disabled due to pneumoconiosis, a substantial set of obstacles was encountered. Some of the testing of pulmonary function involves physical exertion by the claimant. For some of these people, they and/or their physicians believed that such effort could not be safely undertaken due to the claimant's condition. Other tests depended on the individual's complete cooperation. Halfhearted effort could lead to test results similar to those found where there was severely impaired lung function.

Blood gas testing has remained a problem over much of the life of the program. Facilities that could accurately assess the ability of the individual to move oxygen from the lungs to the blood were scarce or unavailable in many of the mine regions. The inability to administer this test to many applicants was given as one reason why ventilatory function test standards should be set at liberal levels, i.e., allowing larger numbers of applicants to be compensated.

The most critical issue of evidence dealt with the X-rays used to determine the presence of pneumoconiosis. It was noted earlier that substantial problems arose due both to the poor quality of many of the X-rays used and to the interpretation of the X-rays. The "B" reader program developed by Johns Hopkins University and NIOSH was designed to overcome these difficulties. Routinely, X-rays that had been interpreted by physicians in the field were sent to "B" readers for a rereading. These "B" readers found very large numbers of errors, based on misreadings by field readers or readings of such poor quality films that no interpretation was possible. (See table 3.1.)

While this sort of scrutiny could be considered laudable under most circumstances where it did not substantially delay the process, it created special difficulties in the black lung program. The overwhelming type of error found by the "B" readers was one where the field readers incorrectly reported the presence of pneumoconiosis. Though Congress had reduced the significance of the *negative* X-ray in the 1972 amendments, positive X-ray evidence of the presence of pneumoconiosis was extremely helpful to claimants, especially after 1972. Program supporters were angered to learn that the "B" readers were undermining claimants who might have been told by a local physician that their X-rays demonstrated the presence of pneumoconiosis. Presumably, some miners had had their expectations raised that they would be entitled to benefits, only to have them cruelly dashed by some distant unknown "B" reader.

The Senate and House chose to take somewhat different routes in dealing with the rereading problem. At the time of the 1977 amendments, the House bill required the Secretary of Labor to accept the opinion of the claimant's physician regarding the miner's X-ray, unless the Secretary had good cause to believe that the X-ray was of unreadable quality or was being fraudulently represented. It is noteworthy that this could have caused some claimants to be denied compensation in those rather rare instances where the "B" reader, unlike the initial reader, found pneumoconiosis present. It also seems striking that the House version did not impose any type of quality control on the claimant's physician, that is, the local doctor could have been a dermatologist by specialty or without any special training in any field of medicine, much less in radiology or chest diseases.

The Senate version provided that where a miner had worked 25 years or more in the mines, and where other evidence existed of pulmonary or respiratory impairment, the Secretary of Labor was required to accept the interpretation of the X-ray given by a board-certified or board-eligible radiologist, if the X-ray was of adequate quality and was taken by a qualified individual, and if there was no reason to believe that the claim was fraudulently misrepresented. The Senate version of this provision was adopted. However, the House conferees were able to drop the Senate's requirement that eliminated the rereading only in cases where miners had worked 25 years or more. (Section 413(b).)

This amendment essentially eliminated the role played by the "B" readers where there was "other evidence" that a miner had a pulmonary or respiratory impairment. The conferees actually went beyond that by inserting in their report: "In the case of X-rays read by a board-certified or board-eligible radiologist, it is the intention of the conferees that the Secretary shall accept, for whatever evidentiary value X-rays generally may have, the evaluation of such X-rays read by a board-certified or board-eligible radiologist without submitting them to a further rereading."[31] The new administration supported the principle of rereading X-rays, but the Congress simply rode roughshod over the position taken by Donald Elisburg, the Assistant Secretary for Employment Standards in the Labor Department.[32]

Though substantially reduced, the role of the "B" reader was not fully eliminated by the 1977 amendments. Before an X-ray report was used as evidence in a claim, a "B" reader had to determine that it met evidentiary standards. The claims examiner in the Labor Department had to accept the "B" reader's findings as to the acceptable quality of the film. If the film was of acceptable quality, taken by a registered radiographic technician (as of March 31, 1980 and later, but waived for X-rays taken before that date), and read by a board certified or board-eligible radiologist, the interpretation had to be accepted as valid X-ray evidence. When the "B" reader evaluated film quality, he was permitted to read the X-ray, but if there was a conflict in interpretation, the one most favorable to the claimant was to be used.[33] Where there were multiple X-ray reports and some were in conflict, doubt was resolved in favor of the claimants. A responsible coal mine operator was free to challenge the X-ray finding and to ask for additional X-ray examination.

As a matter of practice, the administrative law judge placed greater weight on the X-ray most recently taken. In claims involving the Trust Fund, there was no challenge to X-ray evidence presented by claimants where the film was judged to be of acceptable quality by the "B" reader. Section 413(b) was changed in the 1981 amendments so that the prohibition on rereading of X-ray films was removed, except for claims filed before the effective date of the law, January 1, 1982.

When the Labor Department determines that medical evidence is needed to determine the compensability of a claim, the miner is sent a letter with the name of a local doctor who is to examine him. The claimant can use this doctor if he wishes, but has the right to request that his own physician be used. The Labor Department is not required to permit the latter doctor to conduct the physical or X-ray examination, but it generally has allowed this. Individual physicians in the mining areas soon developed reputations as being sympathetic to or tough on claimants. With some choice in the matter and with the predilection of some physicians well known, the quality of physician reporting has been suspect throughout the life of the program.

Where doctors are thought to be biased, the Labor Department's procedures allow it to order an independent examination. In practice, such independent review has not been utilized by the Department.

The role of the examining physician is extremely important in determining the outcome of the claim: "The reasoned opinion of a physician exercising sound medical judgement carries great weight as medical evidence in a claim. A doctor's reasoned opinion can establish the presence of pneumoconiosis (CWP), total disability due to pneumoconiosis (based on medical criteria), and causal relationships of pneumoconiosis to CME (coal mine employment)."[34] The Labor Department's manual spells out what the physician must do to establish the presence of disease where the X-ray evidence is negative. The physician need only state that he is aware that the X-ray is negative, describe the symptoms and the test results, demonstrate a knowledge of the worker's employment and medical history, and rule out other causes for the miner's condition. This suggests that physicians sympathetic to the position of the claimant can play very instrumental roles in helping the applicant. Where there is a responsible coal mine operator to challenge this position with conflicting medical testimony, the claimant may have some difficulty in winning compensation. Where the responsible operator does not vigorously challenge a claim, or where no challenge exists, as in Trust Fund cases after 1977, the claimant's doctor's evidence is likely to go unchallenged.

Early in 1982, the General Accounting Office (GAO) issued a report that evaluated the Labor Department's decisions based upon a sample of 450 claims.[35] The GAO found that 205 claims (45 percent) had been approved. It argued that only 33 claims had provided adequate medical evidence to allow a positive determination of disability or death due to pneumoconiosis. Virtually all the claims had been submitted prior to the permanent standards being imposed by the Labor Department in 1980. Only 7 of the 172 claims that the Labor Department accepted based upon evidence described as inadequate by the GAO were successful because of the opinion of physicians. GAO does not provide data on the number of other successful claims where evidence was found to be inadequate and where a physician's opinion existed alongside some other medical evidence. In its report on SSA's re-review of denied claims after 1977, GAO reported no instances where physician opinion by itself was sufficient to permit benefits to be awarded.[36]

A number of other sticky issues arose in claims from survivors. A recurring problem that appeared very early in the life of the program was one of survivors being unable to obtain evidence useful to their claims. The problem was especially severe in older cases, since, prior to 1969, few doctors in the United States appeared to diagnose or report the presence of CWP or to attribute death to it. The 10-year presumption (section 411(c) (2)) was partially helpful to survivors, but some survivors apparently found it difficult to establish their claims. As of December 31, 1971, SSA had allowed 71,400 "widows" claims and denied 38,000 others.[37]

To ease the burden of proof for survivors, the 1972 amendments added: "In determining the validity of claims under this part, all relevant evidence shall be considered, including, where relevant . . . his wife's affidavits, and in the case of a deceased miner, other appropriate affidavits of persons with knowledge of the miner's physical condition, and other supportive material." (Section 413(b).)

The intent of this section apparently escaped both SSA and the Labor Department, who rejected claims routinely if there was no other support for them except such affidavits. In the 1977 amendments, Congress clarified what it wanted, which was to strengthen the hand of claimants. The House version provided flatly that where no relevant medical evidence existed in the case of a deceased miner, affidavits were to be considered sufficient to establish eligibility. The Senate version was somewhat less munificent and the Conference Committee settled on: "Where there is no medical or other relevant evidence in the case of a deceased miner, such affidavits shall be considered to be sufficient to establish that the miner was totally disabled due to pneumoconiosis or that his death or her death was due to pneumoconiosis."[38] By adding "or other" to the House version, the Conference Committee provided some opportunity to challenge a claim that was based solely on affidavits where no medical evidence was available. The extent to which challenges arose depended on whether or not a responsible coal mine operator was identified. The Trust Fund was far less likely to challenge survivor claimants than were the mine operators.

The GAO found that affidavits were particularly important in SSA's re-review of previously denied claims after the 1977 amendments.[39] In its sample of 131 survivor awards, 78 claims had disability established *solely* by affidavits. In 43 of these 78 awarded claims, the length of coal mine employment was also established by affidavits. According to GAO, in 68 of the 78 cases, the person signing the statement about the miner's impairment was the party filing the claim and seeking the benefits. In its study of Labor Department claims, however, GAO reported that only 7 claims were awarded benefits based solely on affidavits. The study does not provide information on the instances where affidavits were supported by other evidence, such as a personal physician's letter, that itself might be regarded as soft or questionable evidence.

The 1981 amendments tightened up this provision of the law. Beginning January 1, 1982, affidavits from parties with a financial interest in a claim (survivors) are not sufficient to establish that the miner was either totally disabled or died due to pneumoconiosis. The impact of this change was probably quite small, however, since most of the claims involving death had been filed by the effective date of the 1981 amendments. Moreover, in cases involving more recent deaths, medical evidence was more likely to exist. Additionally, even if a widow's affidavit was no longer determining, friends or fellow workers of the miner or of the survivor who would be willing to supply a supportive affidavit would not be difficult to find.

The 1977 amendments also strengthened the position of survivors in another respect. Section 413(b), emerging from the House bill, required the agencies to accept autopsy reports concerning both the presence of pneumoconiosis and the stage of its advancement, unless there was good cause to believe that it was inaccurate or fraudulently misrepresented. In fact, this was not the way the law has been administered, nor did Congress mean what the amendment said. If taken literally, a negative report by a pathologist would leave the agencies no choice but to deny a claim. In fact, where an autopsy report did not find that pneumoconiosis was present at the time of death, the claim could still have been approved if other supportive evidence was forthcoming. By contrast, where pneumoconiosis was said to have been present, the agency was obliged to accept the finding, unless fraud or misrepresentation were evident.

Dr. W. Keith Morgan, a critic of the black lung program, has testified: "It has been my experience, moreover, that certain pathologists indeed regularly record the presence of complicated coal workers' pneumoconiosis when other pathologists with wider and broader experience have been unable to be certain that the histological specimens come from a coal miner."[40] At a minimum, Morgan's charge indicates something about the lack of certainty inherent in autopsy evidence. Beyond that, it suggests strongly that the integrity of some pathologists is open to serious question.

NOTES

1. The evidence for this assertion is presented in Peter S. Barth with H. Allan Hunt, *Workers' Compensation and Work-Related Illnesses and Diseases* (Cambridge: MIT Press, 1980).

2. A miner with totally disabling pneumoconiosis could have died without having received benefits if (a) he died prior to 1970 or (b) he never filed for benefits, even though entitled to them.

3. *Black Lung Program Manual,* U.S. Department of Labor, February 1980, Chap. 2-1004, p. 3.

4. See *Federal Register,* 20 CFR 718.303 proposal of April 28, 1978.

5. See *Federal Register,* 20 CFR 718.303, February 29, 1980.

6. Claims administration is described in chapter 6.

7. Director v. N. American Coal Corp., 626 F 2d 1137 (1980).

8. Usery v. Turner-Elkhorn Mining Co., 96 S. Ct. 2896, 428 U.S. 1 (1976).

9. See Peabody Coal Co. v. Director, 581 F 2d 121 (1978).

10. Kincaid v. Eastern Associated Coal Co., 5 BRBS 369, 371-72 (1977).

11. Rose v. Clinchfield Coal Co., 614 F 2d 936 (1980). See also Pyle v. Allegheny River Mining Co., 2 BLR 1-1143 (January 29, 1981).

12. See *Black Lung Program Manual*, Chap. 2-1001, p. 8.

13. Bozwich v. Matthews, 558 F 2d 475 (1977).

14. *Black Lung Desk Book*, Benefits Review Board, U.S. Department of Labor, August 1981, v-21.

15. Black Lung Benefits Reform Act of 1975, House Report N. 94-770, pp. 4-5.

16. Ibid., p. 5.

17. Hearings before the Committee on Education and Labor, 95th Congress, 1st Session, March 14-17, 1977.

18. Black Lung Benefits Reform Act and Black Lung Benefits Revenue Act of 1977, Committee on Education and Labor, House of Representatives, February 1979, p. 621.

19. See 20 CFR 727.204.

20. Ibid.

21. *Black Lung Desk Book*, x-6.

22. Section 402(d).

23. *Federal Register*, 20 CFR 725.202(a). A rather lengthy explanation and defense of the presumption by the Labor Department follows the description.

24. See *Federal Register*, 20 CFR, August 18, 1978, section 727.203.

25. Ibid., section 727.202(a).

26. Mark E. Solomons, "A Critical Analysis of the Legislative History Surrounding the Black Lung Interim Presumptions and a Survey of its Unresolved Issues," *West Virginia Law Review*, Vol. 83, Summer 1981, p. 895.

27. *Federal Register*, section 727.203(b).

28. See chapter 7.

29. "Black Lung Benefits: An Administrative Review," *Social Security Bulletin*, October 1971.

30. Ibid.

31. Black Lung Benefits Reform and Benefits Revenue Act, pp. 888-89.

32. His testimony was before the Committee on Education and Labor, House of Representatives, March 17, 1977.

33. *Black Lung Program Manual,* Chap. 2-501, p. 11.

34. Ibid., p. 32.

35. Comptroller General's Report to Congress, "Legislation Allows Authorized Benefits Without Adequate Evidence of Black Lung or Disability," January 19, 1982. This is described further in chapter 7.

36. Comptroller General's Report to Congress, "Legislation Allows Black Lung Benefits to be Awarded Without Adequate Evidence of Disability," July 28, 1980.

37. *Black Lung Benefits Act of 1972,* Second Annual Report on Administration of the Act During Calendar Year 1975, U.S. Department of Labor, July 1976, table 3.

38. Since "such affidavits" refers to the preceding sentence which makes mention of "his wife's affidavits," which was taken from the 1972 amendments, the "his death of or her death" does little to expurgate the sexist language in the act.

39. Comptroller General's Report to Congress (1980).

40. Hearings of the Department of Labor on proposed regulations, June 15, 1978, unpublished transcript.

• 5 •
Coverage and Administration

Coverage

The black lung legislation sought to provide protection to disabled miners or their survivors. Supporters of the law consistently argued that they had left the primary responsibility for compensation of victims of occupational illnesses or injuries to state workers' compensation agencies except for one disease, and the single occupational group—miners. Yet, consistent with the other changes that led to expanding the scope of the law from 1969 to 1981, the meaning of the term "miner" took on broader meaning from 1969 forward.

Coverage under the 1969 act was limited explicitly to *underground* coal miners or their survivors. In large measure, this reflected the view that coal workers' pneumoconiosis was a disease caused by exposure to dust within the mines. In the deliberations prior to the passage of HR 9212 in 1972, Representative Michel (R-Illinois) introduced an amendment to strike the reference in the 1969 law to "underground." Michel argued in the floor debate in the House on November 10, 1971

... the fact of the matter is that we have no idea whether or not those who work only in surface mines can contract the disabling disease. While the very limited prevalence studies conducted by the Public Health Service have shown little incidence of pneumoconiosis among surface miners generally,

141

and no evidence of it among those miners who had worked exclusively above ground, no one has ventured to contend that strip miners are not subject to the disease. On the contrary, it would seem reasonable to assume that those strip miners who have worked in extremely dusty situations—at the tipple, for example—for long periods of time, might be subjected to conditions similar to those which result in the development of black lung among underground miners.[1]

Speaking in favor of the Michel amendment, Representative Railsback, another Illinois Republican, explained: "I know that (Michel) has many strip miners in the district which he represents. There are also many in the 19th Congressional District, which I represent and which happens to be contiguous to that of (Michel). Such strip miners deserve to be protected."[2]

John Erlenborn also spoke in favor of the amendment. His support of it symbolizes the basic dilemma in evaluating its justification. On one side, it is difficult to argue that victims of black lung ought not be compensated simply because their exposure to coal did not arise in underground coal mines. Yet support of the amendment on these grounds quickly leads one to support compensating black lung victims who were employed anywhere that coal dust is found, or for that matter, any person suffering from disabling, occupational diseases generally. The other side of the argument, however, is that black lung disease was rarely, if ever, a consequence of dust exposure outside the underground mines. To the extent that a variety of claimant-supportive rules and presumptions enabled persons to receive compensation where benefits could easily have been denied otherwise, this extension of coverage enlarged the pool of potential applicants far beyond the pool of those who actually had been damaged by the disease.

In 1977, Fairman et al. published a paper describing the incidence of pneumoconiosis in 1,438 surface coal miners in 8 surface mines based on U.S. Public Health Service surveys in 1972-1973.[3] Of these, 59 persons (4 percent) showed roentgenographic evidence of some degree of pneumoconiosis, and only 7 (.005 percent) had films classified as category 2 or higher. Five of the 7 showed large opacities consistent with complicated pneumoconiosis. Of the 7, 5 had considerable work experience in underground mines, 1 worker had pulmonary tuberculosis, and one with no underground experience had worked previously in a coal preparation plant. The incidence of bronchitis was relatively high, but significant airway obstruction was uncommon (below 7 percent) in the nonsmoking miners. In summary, complicated pneumoconiosis was extremely rare in surface miners and virtually nonexistent if one credits the few cases found to the miners' previous work in underground mining or (in one case) in a coal preparation plant. Simple pneumoconiosis was also found to be quite uncommon, especially category 2 or 3. Moreover, the previous work histories of those with simple pneumoconiosis were not described.

That coal workers' pneumoconiosis is rare among those with only surface mining exposures is not surprising. Dust levels in surface mining operations are less than one-half of those found in underground mines.[4]

The distinction between surface and underground mining also appeared in the presumptions. One of the presumptions established by the 1972 amendments, and described in detail in chapter 4, was the 15-year rule, i.e., where the miner has or had disabling respiratory or pulmonary impairment, but where the X-ray evidence is negative, there is a rebuttable presumption of pneumoconiosis where the miner was employed 15 years or more in *underground* mining. However, the 15-year presumption could be employed by claimant surface miners or their survivors, if the miner's employment was "substantially similar" to conditions in an underground mine, i.e., some exposure existed to coal dust (see sec. 411(c) (4)). Clearly, Congress chose to maintain a line separating the underground miners from those employed in surface mining. The line was obviously very thin, however.

From 1972 until the passage of the 1977 amendments, considerable controversy swirled around the parties who administered the law regarding the extent of coverage under the act. Section 402(d) defined a miner as any individual who is or was employed in a coal mine. The regulations added that a miner performed functions in extracting coal or preparing the coal so extracted.[5] This led to a two-pronged test of eligibility that examined the issues of situs and of function. The situs matter itself involved two separate questions: Was there a common law employer/employee relationship and was the employment in a coal mine? Where no employer/employee relationship was found, coverage did not exist. Since self-employed miners or independent contractors were deemed not to be employees, they were not covered by the law during this period. Where a claimant leased a mine from the government, compensation was denied, in part, because he was not an employee.[6] The other question involving situs depended on the miner having worked in a coal mine. The regulations treated the term coal mine in a manner that was identical to the definition found in the original law.

The second test was based on regulations requiring that a miner be someone who performed a function in extracting or preparing coal. Was the employee's activity an integral part of the coal extraction or coal preparation process? The following are examples of functions that the Benefits Review Board has found met this test. Where an employee:

—worked in a mine operator's foundry molding replacement parts for mining machinery;

—was a mechanic repairing and maintaining strip mining equipment;
—supervised a prospecting team;
—was a draftsman;
—was a weightmaster in an office and was required to make occasional visits to the tipple;
—was a federal mine inspector;
—operated a grader maintaining haulage roads at a strip mine.

Claims that were denied by the Benefit Review Board prior to the 1977 amendments, because the work was judged not to be integral to coal extraction or coal preparation, involved work as:

—a training specialist preparing audio-visual material and giving lectures on mine safety;
—a negotiator for mineral rights and as a title searcher;
—a truck driver hauling coal from the tipple to private customers;
—a grocery clerk in a mine store located on the town's main street, one mile from the mine. (The Department of Labor had supported compensation in this case.)

The 1977 amendments to the law extended the scope of coverage considerably beyond the 1972 amendments. First, in defining the word "miner" (sec. 402(d)), "any individual who is or was employed in a coal mine" the term "employed" was replaced by "works or has worked." Through this seemingly minor change, coverage was extended beyond employees, to include the self-employed and independent contractors.

In the 1977 amendments, "in a coal mine" was replaced by "in or around a coal mine or coal preparation facility in the extraction or preparation of coal." The addition of coal preparation facility simply codified what had been included by the Department of Labor in its regulations and practices.

The "in or around" language, however, represented a significant extension of coverage under the law. Further, the definition was expanded so as to provide coverage to workers involved with coal mine construction or transportation in or around a mine. Clearly, Congress sought to extend protection under the law on a much broader scale to cover anyone exposed to coal dust in or near the mines.

As a consequence of the 1977 amendments, five types of work became covered under the law; extraction, preparation, mine maintenance, construction and transportation. Persons performing such work and those who provide necessary support functions and performing work which bears a reasonable and necessary relationship to the overall process are covered. As a measure of the sweep of coverage, the regulations add: "An individual employed by a coal mine operator, regardless of the nature of such individual's employment, shall be considered a miner unless such individual was not employed in or around a coal mine or coal preparation facility." [7]

The Department of Labor deals with the "in or around" provision by adding:

> . . . in or around a coal mine or coal preparation facility includes, in addition to mines and coal preparation plants, the mine or plant offices, storehouses, repair facilities located on, or adjacent to or in the vicinity of the mine property, access roads, refuse banks or dumps resulting from the extraction and/or processing of coal at the site on or near the mine property, adjacent railroad or docking facilities providing access to the mine or preparation plant, and may extend to structures and facilities located at some distance from the actual place of extraction or preparation provided such structures or facilities are used in the extrac-

tion or preparation of coal or are intended to be used in or result from such processes.[8]

The coverage since 1977 of transportation and construction workers has led the Department of Labor to insert its own presumption into the regulations it issued. Before then, presumptions had emerged directly in the legislation, but in the August 1978 regulations to implement the 1977 amendments, the Secretary of Labor added one other presumption. A rebuttable presumption was created that coal mine construction or transportation workers were exposed to coal mine dust during all periods of employment in or around a coal mine or a preparation facility. The burden of proving exposure to coal mine dust thereby shifted from the worker. The responsible coal mine operator or the Trust Fund can rebut this only by showing either that the worker was not regularly employed in or around a mine or preparation facility or was not regularly exposed to coal mine dust in the course of such employment.

In summary, a law designed to provide benefits for coal miners and their families began with coverage limited to underground miners. By legislation and regulation, the concept of what a miner is has been extended well beyond workers in underground mines. That coverage would be extended beyond the form that it took in 1969 is hardly surprising, in retrospect. Carl Perkins made it perfectly evident in the floor debate in 1969 that he would eventually extend it. In late October 1969, speaking of the black lung provisions, he said:

> My only reservations about the provisions in the bill go to what is now obvious from the debate and that is—we have not provided broad enough coverage for those miners who have serious respiratory diseases—nor are the benefits adequate for the miner and his dependents. I fully intend that

the Education and Labor Committee will continue to study this problem and the administration of these provisions to assure that they are effective in meeting the needs.[9]

It is clear that Perkins meant these remarks seriously and that coverage, in several senses of the term as he used it, would be widened eventually. The line has been drawn, however, at that point where the finished coal product, that is, after extraction and preparation, has been shipped to the ultimate customer. Thus, a maintainer of a railroad line running out from a mine was compensated on the grounds that his work was an ancillary activity necessary to the extraction or preparation of coal.[10] Benefits were denied, however, where a claimant was exposed to coal dust while employed for a coke producer.[11] Another claimant was awarded benefits by an administrative law judge in the Labor Department in 1977, based on his exposure while crushing coal for a cement manufacturer. On appeal, the claim was denied.[12]

Claims Administration

Social Security Administration

The passage of the Coal Mine Health and Safety Act forced SSA to develop and place into operation with virtually no lead time procedures to administer an entirely new entitlement program. While the Labor Department had over 3.5 years before it was to receive its first claim, SSA had almost no opportunity to plan how it would operate such a scheme. The advantages that SSA had, however, were that it did have its massive field system in place, and that for a number of years it had administered a disability program, Social Security Disability Insurance. An enormous problem for the agency, however, was the inability to guess how much claims activity might develop under the law and what the pace of the flow of claims would be.

The initial burst of claims was not short of amazing. In the first two weeks of the program, 45,000 claims were filed. During the first seven months of 1970, 190,000 claims were received from miners or their survivors by SSA. As a consequence of the 1972 amendments that extended the time under the Part B program and delayed the time of the Labor Department's Part C program responsibilities, SSA continued to be the recipient of new claims until July 1, 1973. Even after this date, SSA handled new claims in two circumstances. If a miner died prior to January 1, 1974, SSA would process any claim filed within six months of the date of death. Second, SSA handled claims filed by survivors of those who had successfully filed as living miners under Part B, where the survivors filed within six months of the date of death.

Claims filed with SSA could be made at any of the nationwide offices of SSA.[13] The claims process was broadly similar to that used in the disability insurance program. The claim was initially dealt with by a claims or hearing examiner. At this level there was an "initial determination" which could result in the claim being granted or denied. If the claimant was dissatisfied with the initial determination, there would be a "reconsideration" based upon reexamination of the existing administrative record by a different individual from the one making the initial determination. If the claimant was still not satisfied, the next level was a hearing conducted by an administrative law judge. The decision at that level could be reviewed by an Appeals Council which had the discretion to grant or deny a review. The next step of the appeal process, which was rarely employed, was U.S. federal district court.

The claims process at SSA differs in one very special respect from the one found in state workers' compensation systems or in some of the Part C cases. The process used in

Part B claims is nonadversarial. The employer plays virtually no role in the case and the claimant need not be prepared to assert his claim against a party seeking to block the entitlement to benefits. As such, the United Mine Workers of America (UMWA) consistently maintained a preference for the Part B approach to claims over that of Part C, which might involve the presence of a responsible mine operator. The union expressed considerable dissatisfaction with aspects of SSA's administration of its program, but it viewed the adversary process in Part C claims with even more distaste.

Appeals of the initial determination were made by claimants only, and not by the agency. In correspondence with Carl Perkins, Secretary Califano wrote in 1977, "I want to inform you that the Department does not, and has not in the past, appealed approved black lung claims at the initial reconsideration level, and do not plan to do so in the future. However, we will reconsider this course of action if we find over time that hearing decisions contain an excessive number of errors."[14]

Claims processing in SSA eventually was handled speedily. One estimate in 1974 was that claims were processed from filing to completion in approximately 10-12 weeks.

Department of Labor

The Labor Department was not involved in handling black lung claims until mid-1973. A task force set up within the Department to plan for the assumption of responsibilities for the program had projected that the average time needed to process a claim would be 90 days. Later, that estimate would be revised upwards to 180 days. This proved to be completely unrealistic as well. In 1976, another departmental task force reported that a survey of 10,000 claims had found that the average time in processing a case was 630 days.[15]

There were several reasons why the Labor Department found it so difficult to respond to claimants in any reasonable amount of time. Much of the problem was said by the Labor Department to be caused by improper or inadequate claims development by the local SSA offices where the claimants went to file their claims. Much of the time in the 630 days was spent securing the needed medical evidence to allow an initial determination to be made. The task force report should have, but did not place any of the responsibility for the problem on the quality of the staff assigned to operate the program, or on its lack of experience in administering an entitlements program.

Some of the Labor Department's difficulties can be traced specifically to the period immediately after the 1972 presidential election. The newly reelected President Nixon requested that all political appointees make available their resignations to the White House and promptly shocked the Labor Department by accepting almost all of them. The insecurity of the very few remaining appointees was understandable and served as a backdrop to other events related specifically to black lung.

Somewhat earlier, the Labor Department had delivered its request to the Office of Management and Budget (OMB) for new positions to staff the program. OMB personnel ruthlessly cut the request, primarily due to its displeasure with the quality of Labor's justification. OMB's goal was not to cut the request as fully as it had, but to force the Department to better justify its request. OMB was prepared to restore much, though not all, of the original request, once Labor made its case more convincing. OMB and Labor Department personnel even met to work out this familiar bureaucratic game. The argument was then prepared by Labor Department staff. However, the Department's surviving leadership, with a view toward currying favor with the White House in its campaign to rein in federal spending, chose not to forward the appeal to OMB. Indeed as the weeks passed OMB was put into the peculiar position of asking where the Department's appeal of its decision was. However, DOL did not make the appeal and the black lung program began with a skeletal staff.

Aside from these difficulties, the Labor Department discovered that, beginning in January 1, 1974, it had run into a buzz saw in dealing with employers. Unlike the SSA program and the Department's transition program that ended December 31, 1973, here was a situation where employers had to be identified as responsible operators, if possible, and liability assessed against them. This proved to be no easy task.

By December 31, 1976, the Department had approved 3,801 claims where a responsible operator had been identified, yet only 123 of these were being paid. The balance were being controverted by the employer, a testimonial to the reluctance of employers to accept the Labor Department's handling of cases.

The Department's sorry record of administration in terms of the prompt resolution of claims eventually caused it to press for a major personnel commitment from Congress and the Carter White House. The Department's argument was strengthened by the massive task handed it with the 1977 amendments—primarily, the need to re-review the pending and denied claims under Part C and some of those under Part B. When Assistant Secretary Elisburg made a request for a supplemental appropriation to raise his black lung staff from 185 to 843 positions, this represented a massive jump for a single program in one of the smallest cabinet agencies. (Actually, the Department had had authorization to fill 270 positions, but 85 had been unfilled for budget reasons.) This would have added about 350 more claims examiners, 75 new administrative law judges (over the 22 on staff) and 26 new attorneys to an existing staff of 9. Congress granted the full measure of Elisburg's request and in August 1978, President Carter signed the supplemental appropriation giving the Department the funding for the 564 new positions.

At the same time, the Department yielded to the miners and the congressional pressures and established eight district offices and 33 satellite offices, with the bulk of these and the jobs they created, in Kentucky, Pennsylvania, West Virginia and Ohio. Eventually, all claims would be processed in one of these district offices. This, also, created the need for more personnel to process claims.

Focusing on the delays and huge backlog of claims in the Labor Department in 1974-76 is not to expose a poorly managed public program. Instead, it is to serve as a basis for understanding the reaction by Congress and the Department itself to the difficulties involved with the program in the first years.

The Claims Process. Individuals seeking benefits under the Part C portion of the law may file a claim at any of the various Labor Department field stations or district offices or with a local SSA office. Initially, that claim is placed under the control of a deputy commissioner (DC). The DC is a supervisory claims examiner, who is empowered to delegate most of his responsibilities to a claims examiner. The DC has the authority to make "initial findings" concerning entitlements to compensation and medical treatment, to order medical tests, to determine the identity of the responsible operator (RO), to determine the fact of disability or death due to pneumoconiosis, to preside at conferences (see below) and to execute orders for the payment or denial of benefits.

The claims examiner (CE) takes the evidence submitted and develops it where necessary with a view toward establishing whether five criteria are met:

1. The claimant has filed a valid and timely claim.
2. The claimant must have been a coal miner or a survivor of one.
3. The claimant must have or have had pneumoconiosis.
4. The claimant must be totally disabled or the miner have died due to pneumoconiosis.
5. The pneumoconiosis must have arisen out of coal mine employment.

If all five of these criteria are met, in fact or presumptively, the CE must determine the date from which benefits are payable, the amount and to whom benefits are payable, and who is responsible for payment.

Miners submitting claims are eligible to receive complete pulmonary examinations at no cost. Appointments are scheduled for consenting miners with physicians located within 50 miles of the miner's home. While reluctant to depend upon the miner's personal physician, the Labor Department will pay for examinations by such doctors, depending upon the physician's specialty and location.

The DC or CE is supposed to notify the potential responsible operator who may be liable as soon as the claim is filed. Where a claim that was denied prior to March 1, 1978 was re-reviewed under section 435, the operator was notified at the time an initial finding was made. The operator has 30 days in which to respond. If the operator accepts identification as the potentially liable operator, it must develop its evidence promptly. The operator has the right to have the claimant examined by a physician it chooses, and the miner must cooperate in the operator's efforts to develop evidence. In practice, the operator may not have scheduled the physical examination until after an initial finding in the claimant's favor, partly as a way to avoid incurring an unnecessary medical expense.

If the initial finding is that there is an entitlement and the responsible operator is identified, the operator has three possible responses. The operator may (1) send the Labor Department an agreement to pay, (2) provide a notice of first payment, or (3) choose to controvert. If the operator does choose to controvert and begins to develop evidence, the claimant may also add evidence to the file to support the claim. When both sides have submitted their evidence, the DC has three options available. The DC may schedule a conference for the parties in order to resolve the issues in dispute. This is usually done within 60 days of the submission of all evidence. If the DC believes the conference will not serve a useful purpose, he may simply approve the claim and issue an "initial determination." Finally, the claim may be denied by the DC and a proposed "decision and order" is issued.

The DC presides over the informal conference. No transcript is prepared and the DC aims to have the parties reach a voluntary resolution of the issues. If the claimant is not represented, the DC must advise the miner or survivor of their rights under law. New evidence usually is not introduced at such conferences.

The "initial determination" is significant inasmuch as the 1977 amendments required that benefits must be paid to the claimant within 30 days of the initial determination. If the responsible operator does not agree to make such payment, the Trust Fund must do so, possibly to be reimbursed at a later time by the RO, with an interest penalty as well. If the claim is denied by the DC, reasons for that are given to the claimant. The miner or survivor has 60 days in which to respond to the denial.

Subsequent to the DC's decision on the claim, either party may request a formal hearing. A request for such a hearing cannot be denied. The formal hearing is conducted by an administrative law judge (ALJ). Each hearing is *de novo* and the DC's findings on contested issues are not considered. The ALJ has the sole authority to determine the issues to be considered and the evidence to be admitted. Within 20 days after the hearings end, the ALJ issues a "decision and order," giving findings and an order. The "decision and order" becomes final within 30 days of its issuance unless it is appealed. The appeal may be either a motion to reconsider or an appeal directly to the Benefits Review Board (BRB). Unless the ALJ's decision is stayed pending the appeal, the responsible operator must begin payments—if found liable—even as the appeal awaits action by the BRB.

Any party in interest dissatisfied with the ALJ's "decision and order" may appeal to the BRB, which derives its authority from section 21(b) (3) of the Longshoremen's and Harbor Workers' Act. This section authorizes the BRB to hear and determine appeals on matters that raise a substantial question of law or of fact. It reviews the case record as well as briefs and memoranda submitted by the parties. No new evidence is introduced and no testimony is heard. The BRB is able to find facts as well as to consider questions of constitutionality.[16] A party adversely affected by the BRB may seek review in the U.S. Circuit Court with jurisdiction for the area where the miner was last employed. As of mid-1981, the average time between a filed appeal with BRB and a decision was about two and one-half years.

In approved claims involving alleged responsible operators, the controversion rate was estimated to be about 90-95 percent during most years of the Part C program. Reasons for the high rate of controversion can be found at several levels. In a Labor Department survey of 10,000 claims, the four principal reasons why cases were referred to ALJ's were disputes over:

1. The existence of pneumoconiosis.
2. The causal relationship.
3. The issue of total disability.
4. The named employer as the responsible operator.[17]

At a different level, reasons for the high controversion rate by employers were enumerated by John Kilcullen, an attorney for several large mine operators, in his testimony on behalf of the National Independent Coal Operator's Association.[18] First, he argued that the 550 pages of administrative regulations issued regarding black lung made controversy a likely outcome. Some of his clients were first notified of claims made against them in 1973 or 1974 as late as 1977. Frequently, he argued, the employers' first notice that there was a claim involving them might have occurred after an initial determination was made (and payment begun). This matter was contested and in 1979, the Fifth Circuit Court upheld the procedures whereby the Department had notified the responsible operator only after the claim had been developed and an initial determination of entitlement had been made.[19] The court found that the Department's procedure did not violate the operators' due process rights.

According to Kilcullen, some operators were forced to controvert as the only way for them to obtain any information about the claim or the basis for the granting of benefits. These employers might then wait months or even a year or more to learn that the matter had been referred to a hearing officer. But Kilcullen also implied that many employers controverted what they regarded as the unjustified granting of benefits to persons not disabled due to pneumoconiosis.

Finally, employers could have resisted paying claims so long as the constitutionality of various portions of the law was in doubt. To do otherwise might have meant making payments to miners and survivors that would not have been recoverable, effectively, at a later time.

The success rate of operators in appealing claims is unclear. Various estimates exist, generally ranging in the 10 percent range, of the operator appeals upheld by ALJ's. In a prepared statement by the United Mine Workers at public hearings in 1981, it was estimated that 10-15 percent of the cases controverted by RO's were overturned and that claims controverted through the ALJ level resulted in employers being successful about 30 percent of the time.[20] These estimates were immediately disputed by Mark Solomons, a former Labor Department attorney who had become a defense attorney retained by some coal mine operators. According to him, an appropriate range for reversals obtained by RO's was about 35-60 percent. "One major coal mine operator has a reversal rate of 78 percent."[21]

One rather direct, if not arbitrary and potentially unconstitutional, manner for dealing with employer controversion appeared in the House version of the 1977 amendments. It provided, quite directly, that no coal mine operator could participate in the adjudication of any claim. The provision was not retained by the Conference Committee.

In contrast to the claims where liability was assigned to an operator, claims were not appealed by the Trust Fund. Indeed, it is the Secretary of Labor only, and neither the Trust Fund nor an employer, who can defend a claim that involves the Trust Fund. In practice, where a claim was granted at any stage of the claim process, initially or on appeal, there would be no appeal by the Secretary to seek to deny benefits, comparable to the practice in SSA under the Part B program. In the light of the employers' ability to successfully controvert initial findings or initial determinations, the absence of appeals by the Secretary or the Trust Fund was especially disturbing to some, including John Erlenborn. Yet the Reagan administration explicitly rejected as unnecessary giving the Trust Fund the right of participation and appeal, arguing that the claims approval rate by late 1981 had fallen to the range of 10-12 percent.[22] Moreover, Secretary Collyer forecast that the proposed amendments would cut this acceptance rate in half, further reducing the need for the Trust Fund to defend itself. The point remains, however, that an active defense by or of the Trust Fund between 1978 and 1981 would have obtained some reversals of entitlements likely in the same general range that operators were being successful in their appeals of claims. Indeed, knowing that claims involving the Trust Fund would not be appealed, while those involving responsible operators probably would be challenged, the Labor Department staff might have been somewhat more lenient in claims involving the Trust Fund.

Aside from the strong likelihood that some benefits were awarded where a defense of the Trust Fund would have led to denials, there were several other costly aspects of the Department's method of administering claims. For one thing, the Department found it difficult to identify where other offsettable payments were being made to beneficiaries. As such, it was widely understood that overpayments were being made to miners and survivors who did not notify the Labor Department of their circumstances. On this point, John Erlenborn testified: "I asked the General Accounting Office some years ago to examine how many workers may be drawing state as well as federal black lung benefits. The answer was that nobody had ever looked, neither social security nor the Department of Labor, and they were not certain that they had a method to find out who was drawing illegally these double benefits."[23]

Additionally, a very large problem revolved about the payments to claimants where an operator's appeal led to a subsequent denial of the claim. Since many of these claims might have involved benefits to be paid as of a much earlier date, a large payment would have been made shortly after an initial determination of entitlement. Lump sum retroactive benefits of $10,000 or more were commonplace. The practice and amounts became especially significant when denied or pending claims were re-reviewed because of the 1977 amendments. Many of these were first filed years earlier, and retroactive benefits were paid if the claim eventually was approved. The essential problem was that once a payment was made, the Department was hard-pressed to recover the money if the claim was subsequently denied. In practice, the Department made very little effort to recover these moneys until recent years, putting virtually no staff into the process.

The Department of Labor had few options as to how it would deal with the problem. It was being subjected to considerable public criticism regarding the delays in its processing of claims. Congressmen from the mining regions were swamping the Department with inquiries regarding the status and circumstances of constituents' claims. Once an initial determination was made, the appeals process could drag on for months or years. Claimants were unable to understand why the granting of a claim left anything to be resolved, particularly since Part B had not involved any such delays or subsequent dispute. The 1977 statute required that prompt payment be made after initial determination of entitlement, though the Labor Department might have been able to delay making initial determinations in the process itself. Where the Labor Department made some efforts to recover payments due to claims reversals, errors in benefits computation, duplicate payments, or the death of a miner or change in someone's entitlement status, complaints to Congress followed. In turn, the Department was accused of harassing widows and disabled miners. Simply in terms of the pressures coming from the legislative branch, the Department had no incentive to seek vigorously to recover overpayments. Moreover, it was easy to rationalize such practices by arguing that the money had already been spent and could not be recovered, no matter how energetically the matter was pursued.

Aside from the revenue implications, this practice weakened the integrity of the claims process. There was a view that ALJs might be reluctant to reverse decisions where benefits had been granted and paid already. To do so, it was argued, would have been simply *pro forma,* as the money was not recoverable. Moreover, that would have left the Trust Fund with the payment since the responsible operator's appeal had been successful. The Department, however, has denied that the appeals process was affected by the payments procedure.

The 1981 amendments sought to end the practice. The Trust Fund is no longer obligated to pay retroactive lump sum benefits where an initial determination of entitlement is made but where the operator contests the award.

An evaluation of the performance of the Labor Department in administering the black lung program depends both on the criteria employed and the vantage point of the evaluator. The Department has received very harsh criticism from both the employer and the labor sides, with additional displeasure registered by Congress, the GAO and even groups inside the Department.

The basis for much of the criticism has been described above. In the earlier years of the program, the delays and enormous backlog were the single most visible aspect of the program to the critics. Promptness of payment or claim rejection, long a bellwether of well-managed workers' compensation programs, was a test that the Labor Department badly failed, whatever the ultimate source of the difficulty.

From the vantage point of the miners and their spokesmen, the Labor Department was seen as too strict and unsympathetic an administrator. Testifying in 1978, a UMWA official said that the union had preferred never to have the black lung program move out of SSA and to the Labor Department. In part, this was because it made the program too much like a workers' compensation program and subjected claimants to an adversary process. Beyond this, however, was the Labor Department's handling of the claim. "The DOL thus far has administered the black lung program with a restrictive vengeance rarely encountered elsewhere. It is punitive to require more than 600 days for processing a claim."[24]

Prior to the enactment of the 1977 amendments, Congressman Perkins described the Labor Department's administrative procedures as "outright discrimination" against the claimants.[25] His assertion was in response to a witness' description of the adversary process employed in Part C claims.

For the administration that ran the Labor Department from 1977 through 1980, the goal was to reduce the enormous disparity between claims entering the system and case closings. This has been spelled out unhesitatingly and without equivocation by Department spokesmen: "It is important to point out here that part of what the Department of Labor has been trying to do the last two years is to get out of this enormous backlog of cases. In less than two years, we have decided over 300,000 cases, and we process them at something close to 3,000 decisions a week to get this monstrous backlog which has been clogging this system for over a decade into a manageable process. I think we are doing that, and that is why you see cases moving into the system and into the Trust Fund process."[26]

The obvious question that follows is, to what extent did this very large movement of claims come at the expense of errors in claims outcomes? A report issued in September 1981 by the Labor Department's Inspector General's Office addresses this directly:

> We recognize that program personnel have been attempting to resolve an extremely large backlog of claims, generated by recent changes to the enabling legislation. However due to the fact that so many of the identified losses could have been easily detected and prevented, without extensive or sophisticated technical resources, we contend that there is clearly a need for better balance between program production and program integrity.
>
> We stress that although substantial loss and loss vulnerabilities within the payment systems have been identified, our greater concern related to the Division of Coal Miners' Workers' Compensation almost total lack of historical interest in and commitment of resources to the prevention of losses, and causal factors and implications of such inadequacy.
>
> In our view, since the passage of the Black Lung Benefits Reform Act of 1977, the Employment Standards Administration and Division of Coal Miners' Workers' Compensation Management have treated the rapid processing of claims and the efficient, responsible management of financial resources as mutually exclusive objectives, and have focused available resources on the processing of claims and delivery of payments.

Finally, the Inspector General cited the agency's failure to move expeditiously to correct known

problems in finding, ". . . major historical and
continuing overpayments generated by faulty and
inadequately designed and implemented payment
procedures and systems, is a clear failure to fulfill
elementary management responsibilities.[27]

Responsible Operators

At the beginning of 1974, coal mine operators assumed
financial liabilities for miners who were disabled or deceased
due to black lung. For a variety of reasons, identification of
responsible operators was no simple matter for the Department of Labor. First, the nature of the industry's labor
market is such that workers frequently change jobs. Compounding this was the reality that so many claims under Part
C stemmed from mine employment that ended many years
earlier. A further complexity was the frequent turnover of
ownership of particular mines, along with the leasing of
mines from owners who did not operate the mine or employ
any miners. Self-employment of miners complicated matters
further. It is not surprising that by the time of the 1977
amendments, DOL was unable to identify a responsible
operator in 75-80 percent of the claims filed under Part C of
the law.

The 1977 amendments that created the Black Lung
Disability Trust Fund helped to clarify, if not eliminate,
some of these issues for DOL. Our focus here is on the identification of the liable party since 1978. Responsibility for
identifying a particular employer as the responsible operator
rests with the claims examiner. Where the claims examiner
encounters any difficulty in making this identification, the
matter is passed on to a "Responsible Operator Section"
that makes extensive use of state regulatory agency records,
Bureau of Mines Legal Identity Reports or private sector
market sources such as Dun and Bradstreet.

The Trust Fund takes liability in claims where a miner's last coal mine employment ended prior to January 1, 1970. This represented a significant change in the law inasmuch as financial responsibility for claims was previously based on the date the claim was filed and not on the date of last employment. The Trust Fund also takes liability for claims involving employment subsequent to January 1, 1970 where the DOL does not identify a responsible employer. Thus, the government was able to shift some financial liability to the coal industry, which was paying for the Trust Fund, and away from itself, even where it could not place the burden on a specific employer.

In defining a responsible operator, DOL extends several tests. First, it defines a *coal miner operator* as:

> . . . any owner, lessee or other person who operates, controls, or supervises a coal mine or any independent contractor performing services or construction at such mine. In accordance with Sections 402(d) and 422(b) of the Act, certain other employers, including those engaged in coal mine construction, maintenance, and transportation, may also be considered to be operators for purposes of this part. An independent contractor or self-employed miner, construction worker, coal preparation worker, or transportation worker may also be considered a coal mine operator. Any employer of a miner may be considered a coal mine operator, based on the circumstances in the particular case.[28]

For a coal mine operator to be deemed a responsible operator, a variety of conditions must be met. First, the miner's disability or death must have occurred, in part at least, as a result of employment by that operator. In a situation where a claimant was employed by a coal mine operator (and other tests are met), there is a rebuttable presumption that the employee was regularly and continuously exposed to dust during his employment with the employer.[29] An employer may successfully rebut this by proving the employee was not exposed to coal dust for significant periods during his employment.[30] An employer was able to rebut this presumption, thereby avoiding liability, by showing that the claimant suffered from complicated pneumoconiosis prior to his first employment with the employer.[31]

A second necessary condition to be established is that the employer must have operated a coal mine after June 30, 1973, the period when the interim Part C program began. Where this condition is not met by the operator, DOL must identify another responsible operator or assign liability to the Trust Fund.

A third test consists of two parts. The employee must have been employed by the (potential) responsible operator for at least one year. By regulation, DOL has determined that one year means 125 days of work. Further, the one year can have occurred over any period of time, e.g., only 25 days employed each year for the past five years. Aside from the one-year minimum employment criterion, the miner also must have worked for the operator at least one day after December 31, 1969.

A final criterion for designating an employer as the responsible operator is that the employer must be capable of assuming liability. According to the regulations, this can be established where there is insurance, including self-insurance, where the firm has sufficient assets to assume potential costs of liability, or even where the operator has an existing business. If none of these is demonstrated, the operator may avoid being identified as the responsible operator, but may be subject to penalties for failure to insure under the act.

The criteria listed above could conceivably be met by more than a single operator in a specific claim. The Labor Department's practice is to assign liability to the most recent of the employers meeting these essential qualifications. Generally, if the mine ownership changes hands, which appears to occur frequently in this industry, liability moves with it to the successor operator. The 1977 amendments changed this in one respect. Where a mine operator, assuming all other criteria are met, sells the mine where the disabled or deceased miner was employed, liability is retained by that operator if the employer remains as an operator in the coal mining industry. Where that condition is not met, the successor operator is liable for the costs of the claim.

Identifying a responsible operator may involve some difficulties for the DOL in establishing the facts involved. For example, to find a *cumulative* year of employment may require delving into some ancient history. Further, the responsible operator may not sit still while being so designated, particularly when another operator may be shifting the burden away from itself. The temptation for the agency is to shift the liability to the Trust Fund, avoiding the controversy but not jeopardizing the claimant's rights to compensation. Indeed, the claimant will face less of an adversary situation where the Trust Fund has potential liability than where a mine operator (or its insurance carrier) is the potential source of benefits. While the temptation may be strong to pursue this path of least resistance, the DOL has made it clear to its Deputy Commissioners that "it is the intent of Congress that liability for payment of benefits be assigned to a coal mine operator whenever possible."[32]

The lines demarcating the liability of a responsible operator (and its insurer), the Trust Fund, and the U.S. Treasury through either Social Security under Part B or DOL for some Part C claims were not always clear. Aside from the obvious confusion that this generated for all the parties concerned, the 1977 amendments created a subsequent furor with a seemingly innocuous change in the law. The 1977 law forced a review of all previously pending or denied claims. This included claims filed between January 1, 1970 and June 30, 1973, which were, of course, claims filed under Part B for benefits from SSA. The 1977 amendments caused the date of application for reopening to be considered as the filing date of the claim. As such, this made these former Part B claims to be Part C claims and the responsibility of mine operators and their insurers or the Trust Fund. Of course, mine operators were liable only if the criteria described above were met, including the one stipulating that the claimant be employed for at least one day after January 1, 1970. Approximately 8,000–10,000 claimants who were awarded benefits under this review, had been turned down originally under Part B, and now became the burden of responsible operators.

Congressman Perkins introduced HR 7745 in the second session of the 96th Congress to shift these claims to the Trust Fund. Congressman Erlenborn expressed suspicion that the motive behind the Perkins move was that the Trust Fund was less likely to controvert a claim than was a private employer. Not surprisingly, the UMWA was a major supporter of the bill. When the Act was amended in 1981 the insurance industry effectively rallied behind this provision, and benefits were made the liability of the Trust Fund and not of the individual operators—and their insurers.

This change ended a potentially nasty battle that was brewing over who had liability in these cases. Insurers had no intention of paying claims against their insureds when they had collected no premiums for this.[33] Mine operators were not readily prepared to accept financial responsibility fully and let insurers off the hook. Ultimately, as a Trust Fund liability, the coal industry had to pay, even though the claims originally had been the responsibility of the federal government.

Statutes of Limitation

One of the serious barriers to compensation for victims of occupational disease can be a statute of limitation. In state workers' compensation laws, a variety of such rules has served to deny potential claimants an opportunity to be compensated.[34] The three most common types of these barriers are the recent exposure rule, the minimum exposure rule, and the filing date-disability rule. The first such limit bars certain classes of claims, often involving pulmonary-respiratory illnesses, where the employee has had no occupational exposure to the hazard in question for some period of time. The minimum exposure rule requires that the worker has spent sufficient time—usually measured in years or shifts of work—being exposed to the hazard in question. Short of meeting this minimum, the claim would be barred. The last rule stipulates that the claim for compensation must be filed within some time period after the disability began, or after the worker knew or should have known of the disability, or some variation of this.

Statutes of limitation or other time-related barriers to filing claims can pose serious difficulties for the claimant, particularly in the case of long-latent diseases. Under the black lung law, however, minimum exposure and recent exposure concepts do not serve to bar any claims. Instead, where they are found (as for example in sections 411(c) (1), (2), (4) and (5)), they serve as criteria for allowing the claimant to invoke presumptions that ease the burden of proof. As such, the recent exposure or minimum exposure usage under black lung is not similar to the application found in certain state laws.

The 1969 law, which was unchanged in this respect in the 1972 amendments, did contain a restrictive statute of limitation. Specifically, it required that any claim for benefits under Part C be filed within three years of the discovery of total disability due to pneumoconiosis or, in the case of a death claim, within three years of that occurrence. (Given the temporary character of Part B, there was no need for a statute of limitation under the Social Security Administration portion of the law.) The law created a special difficulty for widows in some of the older cases that were filed as Part C claims. The Department of Labor estimated in 1977 that 90 percent of the survivors' claims denied until then had been barred by this statute of limitation, and not by any review of substantive evidence.[35] In fact, the statute of limitation was probably more important even than this record of denials suggests, since some widows probably submitted no claims due to this barrier.

The 1977 amendments made three significant changes in the law with respect to the time limitation on the filing of claims. First, the three-year time limit on filing for survivors was eliminated. Thus, there is no longer any statute of limitation in death claims. Second, in the case of claims by living miners, a more liberal rule was enacted allowing claims to be filed within three years of a medical determination of total disability due to pneumoconiosis, or within three years of the effective date of the amendments (March 1, 1978), whichever was later. As such, no claim filed by a living miner until after March 1, 1981 could be barred by a statute of limitation.

The final change in the 1977 amendments eliminated a specific time-based barrier to miners or survivors seeking to invoke the section 411(c) (4) presumption (the 15-year presumption). This change simply widened the applicability of the presumption.

The Department of Labor regulations, as adapted from section 20 of the Longshoremen's and Harbor Workers' Compensation Act, establish a rebuttable presumption that every claim for black lung benefits is timely filed. (See 20 CFR 725.308(c).) The regulation adds, however, that the time limits on filing are mandatory and cannot be waived. The import of these two rules is that where any dispute occurs regarding a possible late filing, the burden of proof rests with the Trust Fund or the responsible operator to show that the claim is not timely.

Attorney Fees

The manner and substance of employee representation under the black lung law have not been without controversy. Some attorneys and other worker representatives, including officials of Black Lung Associations, have purportedly made very large sums of money under the program. Some interviews with persons close to the program reveal a view that for little more work than preparing claim forms for miners or their survivors, and by doing this in volume, some individual representatives have collected hundreds of thousands of dollars in fees per year. This section describes the process of setting and paying legal fees for claimant representation. There are no special procedures in place with respect to fees for defense representation.

There is no requirement that a claimant's representative be an attorney. Where the representative is not an attorney, the adjudication officer, where one is involved, must give approval of the individual designated. Fees to representatives are set by the appropriate adjudication officer (or by the Benefits Review Board). Any prior agreement or contract between the claimant and the representative regarding fees is not valid since the fee is set by the adjudication officer when the claim is resolved. Fees are awarded only where a claim has been prosecuted successfully. The claimant will not pay a fee for legal services where a claim is rejected and there are no benefits granted.

In the 1972 amendments to the Longshoremen's and Harbor Workers' Compensation Act, Congress adopted the principle that the attorney's fee could be added on to the claimant's award.[36] In terms of representation, those provisions have been incorporated into the administration of the black lung program. Thus, there are circumstances where the representative's fee is paid by the employer, over and above the benefits payable to the black lung claimant. Essentially, where the employer declines to pay any benefits within 30 days after receipt of written notice of liability, the subsequent fees incurred by the successful claimant are the defendant's liability.

Where the claimant's representative is not an attorney in a controverted case, the fee must be paid out of the claimant's award. The reason for this special treatment of such representatives is that the Department of Labor believes that the language of the Longshore Act imposes it.

Where an attorney's fee for services is set by an adjudication officer, it becomes a lien against the claimant's award unless it is the defendant's responsibility. Where the representative of the claimant is not an attorney, no lien is made against the benefits award. Again, DOL's belief is that the Longshore Act would not allow such a procedure in the latter situation.

At the time the regulations were approved by DOL in August 1978, it was the Department's opinion that the Black Lung Disability Trust Fund was not able legally to pay a claimant's legal fees. This practice has been changed, so that where the Fund does controvert a claim and benefits are subsequently awarded, the Fund is liable for the attorney fees, over and above the claimant's award.

On what basis is the claimant's representation fee set? The regulations provide the following guidelines:

> Any fee approved under . . . this section shall be
> reasonably commensurate with the necessary work

done and shall take into account the quality of the representation, the qualifications of the representative, the complexity of the legal issues involved, the level of proceedings to which the claim was raised, the level at which the representative entered the proceedings, and any other information, which may be relevant to the amount of fee requested.[37]

The DOL acknowledges the policy that rates are not to be set so low as to drive competent attorneys from the field. The adjudication officer may take into account the risk taken by the attorney in representing a claimant where no fee at all would be paid if there are no benefits awarded. Lay representatives of claimants are to receive lower hourly rates than are attorneys. Attorneys experienced and familiar with black lung claims procedures may receive higher hourly rates than those who are less experienced.[38]

Representation fees have been a continuing source of conflict involving DOL, attorneys and employers. In 1980, about 40 percent of the appeals of black lung claims to the Benefits Review Board involved the matter of attorneys fees.[39] It has been the single issue most frequently appealed at this level. Employers and insurers have appealed "add-on" awards to attorneys that they regard as excessive, and the attorneys have been active in appealing claims where DOL has cut the fee the attorney sought to charge.

The attorney fee allowed by DOL is discretionary. If the employer challenges the award, it has the burden of demonstrating that the assessment "is arbitrary, capricious or an abuse of discretion."[40] If the employer fails to object to the fee application before the adjudicating officer, the Benefits Review Board has held that the employer cannot later object or appeal.

Where the attorney's fee is substantially reduced from the requested amount, the adjudication officer must provide sufficient reasoning to support the reduction. If the reasoning is insufficient, the Benefits Review Board will vacate the decision and remand the case for more specific findings. The fee can be reduced through either of two means. First, the amount of time for services may be viewed as excessive. The attorney is required to provide some detail to the adjudicating officer on the hours of each of the services provided. Second, the adjudicating officer may find the hourly rate to be unacceptable, and reduce it. Either or both of these methods have been employed frequently by DOL to reduce fees, and have often been appealed by the dissatisfied attorney. The matter appears to have occupied considerable time and energy of parties in the hearings and appellate processes.

Insurance Arrangements

In order to understand the black lung program, one needs to be sensitive to the ambitious goal set by Congress that provided for private insurance arrangements. Probably aiming at a close replication of existing state workers' compensation laws and the Longshoremen's and Harbor Workers' Act, the Congress permitted coal mine operators to privately insure themselves against claims for black lung. In allowing the operators to choose the method of insurance they wished, Congress opened the door to yet another interest group that could be expected to develop a stake in the program. It also meant that a tangled web of relationships emerged among insurers, state agencies, mine operators, miner representatives and federal authorities.

The Part C program initially made individual mine operators the principal source of money to support benefit payments. With one significant exception, the operators were required to be insured for worthy black lung claims, should they be designated as the responsible operator. Insurance could be secured in one of two ways. First, upon approval of the Secretary of Labor, a mine operator could self-insure. Group self-insurance was also permitted. Alternatively, the operator could purchase black lung insurance in the market place, either from a private carrier licensed by the state to sell workers' compensation in that jurisdiction, or, if available, from a state insurance fund. Operators that did not secure themselves in one of these ways could be subject to a civil action with fines of up to $1,000 for each day of noncompliance, and possible criminal action.

The significant exception to the insurance requirement involved those employers in either the coal transportation or construction sectors. While the law made such employers potentially responsible to pay black lung claims, they are not coal mine operators. As such DOL has no requirement that they maintain black lung insurance, except that they must secure the payments of benefits for specific claims against them at the time they incur a liability.

A recent DOL annual report describing the black lung program summarizes the existing insurance arrangements under the law.[41] There are approximately 4,500 coal mine operators required by the law to maintain insurance. About 90 percent of these operators had secured insurance through either private carriers or a state fund. Ninety-six applications had been authorized for self-insurance covering approximately 200 companies. In calendar 1981, 14 applications were made to self-insure, of which 4 were approved, 2 denied and the remainder were pending at the end of the year.

The provision of black lung insurance has been highly concentrated in the insurance industry. In 1978, a single private carrier, Old Republic Insurance Company, wrote 31 percent of all the insurance policies for black lung written in that year. The next largest private carrier was the Travelers Insurance Company with 7 percent of the policies sold.[42] Almost 90 percent of the coal mine operators that are insured purchase their coverage from only 12 carriers.[43] In Ohio and West Virginia, exclusive state fund states, workers' compensation cannot be sold by private insurance carriers.

Rate-making for black lung is especially complicated because of the multiple sources of benefits. More specifically, the rate applied to the payroll of coal mine operators in different states will reflect the likelihood that a disabled miner or survivor will file a claim initially at the state level and subsequently at the federal level, or in one jurisdiction only. In several instances at the state level, compensation for dust diseases may be partly or fully the liability of a state fund and, hence, not reflected in the premiums paid under a workers' compensation black lung policy. Since benefits paid by such a fund will reduce the operator's individual liability, the premium paid by the operator will be lower, all other things being equal. Since state benefits remain at a constant level once benefits payments have begun, but the federal benefit level is indexed to federal employee salary levels, persons drawing only state benefits or state and federal benefits are expected to depend increasingly in the future on federal payments, raising the potential liability of mine operators and their insurers.[44]

It has been noted that rates on insurance purchased from private carriers vary because of different state practices, e.g., the provision of some or all state benefits through a special state fund, and because of decisions by state insurance commissions in rate filings. Yet another reason for differences is that the rate reflects an estimate of the number of compensable responsible operator claims in the state related to the total number of actived miners in the state. Thus, rates will be higher, all other things held constant, where employment in earlier years was higher—or current levels of mine employment are now depressed relative to former times. Also, rates will be higher where there have been more accepted claims on responsible operators. Numerous claims for black lung involving private insurers have been accepted by the states of Pennsylvania, Kentucky and Virginia, the latter being the only state which typically compensates for partial disability due to black lung. By contrast, Colorado, Illinois and Indiana have regularly rejected most state claims for black lung.[45] The customary policy provided is simply a black lung compensation endorsement attached to a workers' compensation policy. Such a policy protects the operator from claims brought in either the state or federal jurisdiction.

Why did the insurance industry decide to write policies for black lung insurance? In several respects the decision to do so was not a simple one. The industry had virtually no experience in dealing with such a phenomenon as black lung, where the determination of eligibility for benefits was subject to such a high degree of variability, based on shifting policies and politics involving both the executive and legislative branches of government. Further, future benefits under black lung were indexed both in new claims and where benefits had already been established, creating uncertainties as to appropriate reserve practices and rates. And quite unlike virtually all forms of conventional insurance, the insurers were covering a condition that had already existed for many of the prospective claimants. The contingency for which insurance was being sold was not the development of disabling or killing disease, since in most cases these events had already occurred. Instead, the event that was being insured was that a claim would be filed and benefits granted by DOL. This clearly represented an unconventional, insurable risk.

The decision to provide black lung insurance reveals a good deal about the industry's concerns at that time. One industry source who has been very close to this program has explained it in this way:

> First, and perhaps foremost, the federal govern-
> ment was playing a very active role in evaluating
> workers' compensation in 1972. Considerable
> discussion of federal standards for state laws under
> the threat of federal intervention was prevalent in
> 1972. We all know of the 19 essential recommenda-
> tions of the National Commission that set
> minimum standards for state laws and caused much
> state legislative action in the 1970's. The industry
> was looking for a chance to prove its usefulness and
> cooperate with the federal government. We were
> not anxious to see the federal government continue
> as providers of insurance in any form.[46]

The threat to the insurance industry from federal en-
croachment into state workers' compensation programs may
or may not have been real, but Congress had considered the
creation of a federal insurance fund. Indeed, the 1977
amendments created the authority for DOL to establish such
a fund should it find that insurance was not available at
reasonable cost to coal mine operators. At that time the congressional conferees made it clear that such a fund was not to
become a pool for high risk operators, as some state funds
appeared to have become under workers' compensation. If
such a fund were to be created, it was to charge rates consistent with accepted actuarial practices. A federal black lung
insurance fund would have been viewed with concern by the
insurance industry, primarily as it might serve as the vehicle
to expand beyond black lung into other lines of coverage.

Two additional reasons were given for the industry's willingness to underwrite black lung insurance. The industry
thought that the vast bulk of the old claims had been dealt
with under the Part B program, and that they were insuring,
effectively, those miners still employed. Further, the industry believed that rates would be adequate to deal with
eventual claims. "We had the liberty of charging a substan-

tially high rate with a large margin for error. A 40% load was included in the initial rate to handle contingencies. The rates exceeded $25 per $100 of payroll in some states, surely that would be enough."[47]

The process of rate-setting for black lung appears to have been far more complicated than for state workers' compensation schemes. First, while benefits and eligibility criteria are set federally, rates are generally subject to approval by the individual state insurance commissioners. The varying degrees of success in having proposed rates approved by these agencies partly explains the very large interstate differences in the black lung rates being paid by the mine operators.

Table 5.1
Occupational Disease Premium Rates
by Major Coal Producing States, Underground Exposure,
per $100 Payroll, Selective Periods

	Initial rate July 1, 1973	Rate Jan. 1 1980	Rate Dec. 31 1981
Alabama	$25.49	$16.20	$16.20
Colorado	17.33	16.15	16.15
Illinois	26.47	26.47	26.47
Indiana	26.16	16.68	16.68
Kentucky	None	12.12	18.50 (prospective)
Kentucky			34.87 (retroactive)
*Ohio	6.30	6.41	6.30
*Pennsylvania	3.61	7.88	24.72
Tennessee	25.41	16.00	16.00
Utah	28.60	19.49	28.60
Virginia	23.89	16.74	16.74
*West Virginia	7.15	7.15	7.15

SOURCE: Cols. 1 and 2, DOL Annual Report for 1979, p. 37, and Col. 3 from DOL Annual Report for 1981, p. 4.

*Federal black lung increment only.

As noted above, historic data were of no use in the initial rate-making efforts in 1973. By way of reducing the risks imposed on the insurance industry, the 40 percent surcharge was imposed. To further reduce the risks of any single carrier, the bulk of the insurance was placed in reinsurance pools. Estimates of the potential for claims were based in part on NIOSH studies of the incidence of black lung disease.

From 1974 until the end of the decade, insurers found this line of business to be highly profitable. Because of delays in claim processing, along with employer resistance when designated as responsible operators, very few black lung benefits were actually paid to claimants. As Table 5.1 demonstrates, from July 1, 1973 until 1980, the majority of the major coal producing states actually reduced their rates. The industry's windfall ended suddenly in 1979-80 for two reasons, First, the enormous backlog of unresolved claims that had built up in DOL since 1974 had been processed. Partly because of the 1977 amendments liberalizing eligibility for benefits, a significant share of these were accepted and became the responsibility of an insurer. Second, the 1977 amendments allowed for a review of all previously denied claims under Part B and C, swelling further the applicant pool. Many of these claims eventually resulted in employer/insurer liability.

Making matters even worse was the inability of the industry to obtain up-to-date and reliable data on claims and awards, due largely to DOL's inability to develop an effective information system. Operating in the dark, the industry was hard-pressed to evaluate the dimensions of the liabilities it faced. Further, inadequate data meant that evidence could not be developed so as to obtain adequate rate increases in all the various states in which they operated. The industry would have had little problem with a growing liability for black lung, had it developed gradually and in a manner that allowed rates to be adjusted accordingly. Moreover, the earlier experience of considerable profitability from this line may have made the industry's plight less compelling to state insurance commissions.

As noted elsewhere, the industry was also embroiled in a controversy with both DOL and some employers over those reviewed claims that had been initially filed prior to July 1, 1973. While these claims were originally denied under Part B, they became the potential liability of responsible operators after the 1977 amendments. The industry argued that no premiums had ever been paid to provide insurance for these applicants.

The result of the 1977 amendments and the DOL's speed in moving claims was a suddenly dismal condition for the industry. The culmination of all this was two widely circulated reported by a securities analyst spelling out the industry's plight.[48] Emanating from an insurance specialist operating from Hartford, the later report estimated that the industry was seriously under-reserved. Specifically, it estimated that the insurance pool held only $520 million in reserves as compared to a present value of reserves required of from $599 million to $999 million based on a projection of successful claims reported through 1980 (using a discount rate of 3-1/2 percent). On this basis, the pool was under-reserved by somewhere between $79 million and $479 million—in present value terms—which Conning calculated as being 0.6 to 3.4 percent of all earned premiums for workers' compensation in 1980. Conning's report described how this situation had developed so suddenly by pointing out that DOL had approved, overall, 59,425 claims from July 1, 1973 until March 14, 1980, of which 21,919 claims were approved between October 19, 1979 and mid-March of 1980. As opposed to a gradual and easily recognized growth of claims to which the industry (and rates) could adjust, black lung insurers instead were overwhelmed by a tidal wave of claims. The industry's response was to push vigorously for higher rates and to lobby for legislative relief culminating in the 1981 amendments.

The Black Lung Disability Trust Fund

Background

For a variety of reasons, a coalition of the interest groups formed around the concept of a Trust Fund to pay benefits under the Part C program. Legislatively, the origin of such a fund was HR 10760, in the 94th Congress, which passed in the House of Representatives in 1975. This version created an insurance trust with coal operators serving as trustees of the fund. In 1976, the Senate studied a somewhat different version than the one approved in the House in 1975 that used a tax mechanism to support such a fund. The end of the session arrived before the Senate took any final action on the bill.

In the 95th Congress, a Trust Fund bill, HR 4544 cleared the House. A similar bill with a different type of tax from the one approved by the House cleared the Senate in S 2538 resulting, ultimately, in Public Law 95-227, the Black Lung Benefits Revenue Act of 1977.

As noted, support for a trust fund emerged from several sources. In testimony before the House Committee on Education and Labor, Arnold Miller, President of the UM-WA, endorsed a trust fund approach and urged that *all* new black lung claims, where worthy, be compensated from such a fund.[49] His preference for a trust fund approach stemmed from his displeasure with the adversarial approach taken by most of the coal mine operators who were named in specific claims as responsible operators. Miller's aim, quite openly, was to replace the adversarial process by one device or another, and the trust fund would be an acceptable means to accomplish that.

Carl Bagge, president of the National Coal Association, testified at the same set of hearings as Miller and, while not endorsing the trust fund approach, he made precise recommendations as to how the fund should be financed. John J. Kilcullen, speaking for the National Independent Coal Operators Association, endorsed the trust fund as an acceptable alternative, *if* there had to be a federal black lung program. Kilcullen argued that the fund should be used solely where no responsible operator was identified. He also warned that unless approvals for payments were made by fund trustees, presumably coal mine operator representatives, DOL's Office of Workers' Compensation programs would err on the side of excessive generosity in approving payouts from the fund.

The coal mine operators who supported a trust fund believed it allowed for greater certainty or predictability in terms of their costs. From their vantage point, claims had been assigned to individual operators on an almost haphazard basis.

Donald Elisburg, only recently confirmed as Assistant Secretary for Employment Standards in the DOL, testified in favor of using a trust fund. He argued, with Arnold Miller and with Rep. Perkins, that the adversary process was detrimental to the administration of the program, and he seemed to support the possibility of eliminating it entirely.

Overall then, the UMWA and the new Carter administration endorsed some type of trust fund approach, as did at least some significant portions of the coal mine operator community. Additionally, with Perkins solidly behind the idea, and with little opposition save for some warnings by Erlenborn about the potential for abuse, the success of the legislative initiative was assured.

Trust Fund Responsibilities

The Black Lung Disability Trust Fund created under the 1977 legislation was primarily responsible for paying benefits (both medical expenses and cash compensation) to eligible miners and their dependents in two situations. First, it was the source of funds in Part C claims where DOL was unable to identify a responsible operator. Up until then, these claims had been paid out of general revenues; as of April 1, 1978 they would be paid out of the Trust Fund. Second, the Trust Fund was to pay for worthy claims where the last coal mine employment occurred prior to January 1, 1970, i.e., before the Coal Mine Health and Safety Act took effect. With many such old claims still being filed with DOL, along with many others pending determination as to entitlement or liability at the time the bill was enacted, it is clear that these old cases constituted a sizable potential expense for the Trust Fund.

Prior to the 1977 law, Part C claims were to be the liability of responsible operators, where they existed and could be identified, even when the last coal mine employment occurred before 1970. Only a tiny handful of these claims were actually being paid by the operators, who controverted virtually all such claims for old cases. Given the delays in DOL and the Benefits Review Board in adjudicating such claims, claimants were paid by DOL and not by the coal mine operators, at least until liability was resolved on a case by case basis. Since the 1977 law now made the Trust Fund the source of payment for claims based on last coal mine employment prior to 1970, it made sense to no longer extract continuing payment from the few operators who were paying such claims at the time of the amendments. Instead, the law had the Trust Fund reimburse those few operators who already had incurred some expenses in paying for these claims.

The Trust Fund's other financial responsibility was to reimburse the government for payments made under Part C claims between January 1, 1974 and March 31, 1978, along with the administrative expenses incurred by the agency. Based upon these charges and the reimbursement of the coal mine operators who paid claims where the last employment preceded January 1, 1970, the Trust Fund incurred an immediate, one-shot expense of over $90 million, about 30 percent of which represented a repayment of government administrative expenses.

The 1977 amendments required a review of thousands of claims that were pending at that time or had been denied previously by DOL and SSA. Where a Part C claim was found worthy upon review and originated from a last coal mine employment that preceded 1970, this was to be a liability of the Trust Fund. Since such benefits were payable as of the date of filing the claim or January 1, 1974—whichever was later—many of the reviewed claims that were accepted involved sizable retroactive benefit payments in lump-sums to miners of dependents.

A final responsibility of the Trust Fund was the obligation to pay interest charges on any advances from the U.S. Treasury, if and when revenues proved inadequate to meet fund obligations. This, along with the less significant but symbolic charge to the Trust Fund of expenses incurred in program administration, revealed the interest by Congress in pushing as much of the cost of black lung onto the coal industry as possible. To some extent, it reflected congressional anger over the industry's earlier reluctance to accept the financial burdens of the program in the period 1974 to 1977.

Trust Fund Revenues

The decision to create a trust fund that was to be fully paid for by the coal industry must be viewed as a political expedient. If the decision had been instead to tap general revenues, political reaction to the program generally, and the liberalizing amendments of 1977 in particular, would have been more difficult to overcome. By appearing to place the direct burden on the coal industry, Congress seemed to satisfy the traditional conservative goal of "internalizing" to the industry the social costs that emerged from coal production. It also seemed to promote the notion that individual operators might operate less dusty and hazardous mines in order to keep future Trust Fund obligations lower. The Trust Fund satisfied an even vaguer notion that, since the industry had profited in the past from operating disease-producing mines, some punitive action of this sort could be justified.

A variety of problems are involved with each of these views. Yet, the Trust Fund concept, based on a charge to mine operators, can be defended on the most significant grounds of all, that is, in 1977 it was a politically acceptable scheme to fund benefits. In a search for someone to pay for claims emerging from pre-1970 coal mine employment or in the absence of any identifiable responsible operator, the coal industry was an available source of "deep pockets." The industry bore sufficient guilt in the public mind for permitting the disease, and its uncooperative approach until 1977 did little to cast it in a more favorable light.

What are the major objections to a trust fund based on coal industry funding? First, the coal industry of 1978, or of subsequent years, is not the industry of 1969 or of earlier decades. In theory, internalizing costs would force a producer to bear the social as well as the private costs of production. In turn, product prices would reflect the full costs of production, both public and private costs, thereby encouraging users to purchase alternative products that are now relatively cheaper.

These conventional arguments have been used to justify workers' compensation insurance systems.[50] Where they have merit is in cases involving injuries due to accidents. The theory is not acceptable, however, when applied to long-latent occupational diseases that are derived from hazardous exposures of earlier periods. One cannot justify internalizing a cost today, except perhaps in a punitive sense, for a product that was priced and sold 5, 10, or 20 years ago.

As a punitive or socially vindictive approach, the coal industry's responsibility to be the sole source of support for the Trust Fund is equally hard to justify. Many of the coal mine operators of 1978 had not been in the industry at the time that earlier exposures to dust were causing black lung. Many of those operators who had been responsible for dustry or hazardous mines were long since removed from the coal scene. Profits made as a consequence of such practices years or decades ago could hardly be tracked down and reclaimed for such a trust fund. Some of those profits had been distributed to stockholders with little or no long-term commitment to the shares of ownership that they held at one time. Higher profits conceivably helped fuel demands by miners for higher wages and benefits, making them partial beneficiaries of practices that enlarged the profits of earlier coal mine operators. Additionally, if unhealthy mines permitted coal to be sold at lower prices than would have occurred if sanitary and healthful conditions had been maintained, then benefits from such practices also accrued to coal users in the form of lower prices for electrical or heating services, as well as steel and other coal-using products. The failure to internalize coal costs in earlier years when miners were being exposed to coal mine dust meant that the public, consisting of individuals and businesses outside of the coal industry, in those years were beneficiaries also. As such, it seems difficult to justify limiting the financial supporters of the Trust Fund to the existing coal industry of 1978 and beyond, except on the grounds that it would be acceptable politically.

In theory, once the coal industry is identified as the source of funds, there are three possible types of taxes that could be levied. The nature of the coal business is such that there are enormous intraindustry effects of the different types of tax selected.

One approach could have involved a payroll type of tax, with some limited justification based on the notion that the more employees there are in a mine, the higher the potential source of future claimants. This would have moved the funding mechanism somewhat into line with the basis for workers' compensation benefits. Such a tax would be most costly to labor-intensive mining operations, putting them at a competitive disadvantage with more capital-intensive producers. The more labor-intensive mines tended to be in Appalachia, where considerable disemployment had been occurring already, and were also in the areas that were most unionized. Such an approach could be expected to hasten the substitution of capital for labor in the labor-intensive mines or to simply shut them down, a circumstance that was unacceptable both to members of Congress from underground mining regions and to mine workers' unions.

The other two approaches to an industry tax could involve a levy on the sales price of coal, or a tax on the coal tonnage sold. In 1977, the Senate bill provided for the former while the House version created a tax based on the latter. A tonnage tax had a type of precedent with the UMWA health and pension plans having been funded, through collective bargaining, with a tonnage charge.

The significance of each of these approaches derives from the large price differences that exist for coal. Strip mine coal and western coal usually sell for considerably less than do underground mined coal and eastern coal. Coal burned by utilities is of different quality and price than metallurgical coal. Thus the form of the tax can differentially impact various parts of the industry. Examples of this are evident from table 5.2.

Table 5.2
1979 Average Prices, FOB Mine,
per Ton, Excluding Lignite

	Region		
Source	East	West	U.S.
Surface	$22.93	$10.44	$18.66
Deep	33.36	23.53	32.76
Total	28.42	11.97	24.73
*Metallurgical	42.58		
*Steam	17.49		

SOURCE: Provided by the Department of Energy, Hearings before the Subcommittee on Ways and Means, House of Representatives, July 27, September 28, 1981, Serial 97-32, 1981.

*1978

The congressional conferees settled on a hybrid tax that represented something of a compromise in the positions of the two houses. The 1977 act provided for a fixed tax per ton of coal sold, with the rates set so that underground mines paid $.50 per ton while strip miners paid only $.25 per ton. Additionally, if these rates resulted in a tax that would exceed 2 percent of the sales price of the coal, the 2 percent rate would apply.

Another consideration in the method of taxation selected by the Congress involved the nature of sales contracts in the industry. Some coal is sold under long-term contracts to major consumers. An excise tax levied on the sale is (initially) paid by the consumer, while a tonnage tax is paid by the seller. Economists know that the ultimate incidence of the tax may fall on either or both parties to the transaction according to underlying conditions of the supply of and demand for coal. Where there are long-term contracts in place however, and there is no renegotiation of them, a tonnage tax will fall entirely on the coal supplier and not on the purchaser. The mine operator whose coal tended to be sold under these long-term contracts preferred an excise tax approach, but the idea was unacceptable to Congress. The legislators wanted the tax to fall, and appear to fall, squarely on the coal mine operators.

At the time that Congress was considering a change in the Trust Fund coal tax in 1981, one industry spokesman gave the following demonstration of the differential impact of the 1977 tax. Martin White, vice president and general manager of the Western Energy Company, a Montana surface mining company, pointed to the following: for the second calendar quarter of 1981, underground mines produced 10.2 tons/man-day; at $.50/ton, they paid $5.10 tax/man-day.[51] On average, surface miners produced 35.2 tons/man-day and at a rate of $.25/ton, paid $8.80 tax/man-day. In Montana, average surface mining production was 119.6 tons/man-day, at $.25/ton, or a Trust Fund tax of $29.90 tax/man-day. Thus, the Montana operator paid almost six times the tax rate per worker that an average underground operator did, despite the fact that the health risks of underground mining were considerably greater than of surface operations.[52]

Trust Fund Adequacy

In the light of the earlier experience under the black lung program, it was hardly surprising that the Trust Fund's needs were very badly underestimated and, therefore, underfinanced. The Trust Fund's inadequacy stemmed from several sources. The volume of new incoming claims was underestimated, as was the forecast rate of acceptance of new and reviewed claims by DOL. Interest payments to the Treasury to repay advances were required by the statute to be based on market interest rates, and these became quite high after 1977.[53] More important, they were considerably higher than the 6 percent rate charged to coal mine operators who were required to repay the Fund for payments to a claimant. The 6 percent rate was set by DOL regulation.[54] Further, benefits paid by the Fund were indexed and rose somewhat with the inflation rate. The tax, however, being a flat-level tonnage tax, was unaffected by inflation (except as the 2 percent of selling price maximum was affected) and varied only with coal output. Even the absence of recession in 1980-81 would have found the Trust Fund in difficulty, but the economic circumstances of the industry totally undermined the original approach.

The actual experience of the Trust Fund is indicated in table 5.3.

Table 5.3
Black Lung Disability Trust Fund
Fiscal Year 1978-81
(in millions)

Type of obligation and revenue	1978	1979	1980	1981
Monthly benefits	$119.9	$574.4	$707.0	$ 623.2
Hospital and medical benefits		8.7	9.5	37.4
Administrative cost	35.3	32.1	34.2	35.6
Interest charges	0	7.7	52.5	109.5
Total obligations	155.3	623.0	813.2	805.6
Total revenues	93.2	221.7	272.3	236.6
Treasury advances	18.9	400.8	535.8	554.8
Cumulative debt	18.9	419.7	955.6	1,510.3

SOURCES: Adapted from Black Lung Benefits Act, Annual Report on Administration of the Act during Calendar Year 1981, U.S. Department of Labor, Table 4, and Background Material and Dates on Major Programs within the Jurisdiction of the Committee on Ways and Means, 97th Congress, 2nd Session, February 18, 1982, p. 241.

The table shows that the Trust Fund was very badly under-financed in each of the years it existed and that it rapidly incurred a cumulative debt to the Treasury of over $1.5 billion. During this relatively short time period, the Fund had taken in from taxes under $825 million and had expenses of over $2.3 billion. By the end of FY 1981, the Fund was paying almost $110 million/year in interest expenses (roughly 40 percent of revenues) on the debt it had accumulated in under four years of operation. By early 1981, sources in DOL were estimating the future liability of the Trust Fund to be in excess of $6 billion, and there were some private actuarial estimates that were twice as large. Even the smaller number was well in excess of original cost projections. It was clear that steps had to be taken, but the administration chose to delay any move until after the election in November 1980.

A serious issue that the Trust Fund faced was its appropriate role in claims processing. The law creating the Trust Fund gave it no role in challenging Labor Department determinations. Its role had been simply to pay any claim involving Trust Fund liability approved by DOL. Conservatives in Congress, including John Erlenborn, and coal industry representatives urged that the Fund play a larger role than given to it in 1977, that is, to defend itself against claims. Yet liberal support for the Trust Fund and that from the UMWA developed primarily because it avoided an adversarial process for claimants. The worthiness of claims involving the Trust Fund was to be evaluated by DOL, serving as both a fact finder and as a judge. The Trust Fund's financial inadequacy was so overwhelming that no reasonable degree of defense against claims could have kept it out of debt. It is likely, however, that its financial position would have been strengthened, could it have disputed DOL determinations that resulted in obligations for the Fund.

1981 Amendments

The Reagan administration's 1981 amendments to the black lung law contained several important changes involving the Trust Fund. First, as of January 1, 1982, the tax rates were all doubled, i.e., a tax per ton set at $.50 for surface mines, at $1.00 for underground mines, and a 4 percent maximum based on sales price. The increase has been described as interim, since the tax is scheduled to revert to pre-1981 rates on January 1, 1996 or sooner if the Trust Fund pays off all its cumulative debt to the Treasury. It was anticipated that advances from the Treasury would no longer be needed by FY 1984 and that the debt to the Treasury would be repaid entirely by FY 1993.[55] Another source forecast that the Trust Fund would have to continue to borrow until at least 1987.[56]

Whether the tax increase will prove sufficient is not known, but the prognosis is unfavorable.[57] Virtually all projections associated with this program have been badly flawed. Most projections have tended to underestimate future program utilization and costs. A possible exception to this, bearing directly on the Trust Fund, was Assistant Secretary Elisburg's testimony in late 1980 where he forecast that the Fund's costs over its first 20 years would be $20-22 billion, with a Trust Fund cumulative debt of $9.2 billion by 1995.[58] In contrast to these DOL projections, Congressman Perkins and a UMWA official agreed in conversation that the Fund would "come out of the red within the next year and especially two or three years from today, the Trust Fund would be, I would say, within five years, the Trust Fund could easily be solvent, so no one knows for certain, but that could easily be the case with the increased production of coal."[59] This has proven to be unusually wide of the mark in the first 2-3 years of the new tax.

Aside from doubling the tax in 1981, the amendments provided that interest rates charged to operators by the Fund be based on market conditions. This made the rates consistent with those paid by the Fund on its debt to the Treasury.

The 1981 amendments also shifted to the Trust Fund 10,200 accepted cases that previously had been the responsibility of the individual operators and their insurers. These cases, described in more detail earlier, were claims that were initially denied and then approved upon review resulting from the 1977 amendments. The Congressional Budget Office estimated that these cases would increase the Trust Fund's expenditures by over $120 million between FY 1982 and FY 1986, exclusive of the debt service generated by this new obligation. An insurance industry trade association testified in 1981 that the present value of the 10,200 cases, as of that time, was $1.5 billion.[60]

State Laws

The original concept of the black lung legislation was to have the federal government accept the existing pool of potential cases of death or disability due to CWP and, after a transition period, turn claims for currently developing cases over to the states. Subject then only to certain federal standards, the states would incorporate such claims into their own workers' compensation laws.

The state's role in administering and paying for black lung claims was not solely limited to the post-transition period. Section 413(c) of the 1969 law mandated that no claims were to be considered under Part B unless the claimant also had filed a claim under the applicable state's workers' compensation law prior to or at the same time the federal claim was filed. An exception to the requirement was that no state claim had to be made where the filing was clearly a futile matter. Such a case would occur for several reasons, including that the state did not provide for such benefits, or that the timing in the case exceeded some statute of limitation making the particular filing futile.

The plan did not appear to be unreasonable in 1969 or in 1972 in light of what Congress had been led to believe. First, the greatest expense of compensating for black lung derived from disabilities and fatalities that had occurred already and would be paid under Part B of the program. By the time Part C became effective, these claims were to have been resolved and payments made on them by SSA. The view that Part C would not involve many claims was strengthened by a hope that the post-1969 federal dust standards would lead to a lower incidence of pneumoconiosis. Second, most parties involved with state workers' compensation laws, i.e., state administrators, insurers, employers, some health providers, were known to want to retain program administration at the state level. Organized labor was an exception to this, but not uniformly or emphatically so. A federally administered program for compensating an occupational disease was a threat to state sovereignty over such programs, as it represented a possible model for further federal control. Turning such a federal program back to the states appeared consistent with the national movement from a Great Society to a New Federalism, where the latter entailed a return to the states of control that had previously been moved to the central government.

The Secretary of Labor was responsible for certifying that the states met the federal standards so as to move program administration from Washington back to state agencies. Section 421(b) (2) spelled out the criteria by which the Secretary would evaluate state laws so as to assure that they provided "adequate coverage for pneumoconiosis." Essentially, these provisions required that the cash benefits be "substantially equivalent to or greater" than federally provided benefits under Part B, and that the criteria used to determine eligibility be "substantially equivalent" to the federal ones that had been legislated and established through regulation by the Secretary of Health, Education and Welfare.

A number of states made some movements to receive such certification. In 1973, four states—Kentucky, Maryland, Virginia, and West Virginia—submitted plans to the Secretary of Labor. Ultimately, certification was not given, the plans were withdrawn, and the program never was returned to the states. The impediment to carrying out this transfer of responsibility from DOL to state workers' compensation agencies was the requirement that even those newly filed claims based on last employment prior to state assumption be a state's responsibility. Thousands of claims continued to pour into DOL based on last employment dates prior to July 1, 1973, and in many cases much earlier than that, and these would have to be dealt with by state agencies. In many cases, no employer would be found to pay such claims, resulting in a need for the states to raise sizable funds to do so. Ultimately, these "old" cases kept the plan for the assumption of responsibility by the states from succeeding.

The intent of Congress to have the federal government get out of the business of running the black lung program was expressed again in the 1977 amendments. Section 421(b) (2) (A) was amended to allow the Secretary of Labor to certify a state law's compliance with the federal standards where benefits are provided for death or disability due to pneumoconiosis, except that "such law shall not be required to provide such benefits where the miner's last employment in a coal mine terminated before the Secretary's approval of the state law pursuant to this section."

This amendment did not absolve the mine operator of liability for claims where the last employment had occurred prior to the Secretary of Labor's certification. It meant that these earlier cases would be administered by DOL and paid for by either a designated responsible operator or the Trust Fund. The coal mine operator was still required to obtain insurance under the federal scheme and be subject to the tonnage tax that supported the Trust Fund. The 1977 amendment did not succeed in having states seek certification.

In 1981, Deputy Undersecretary of Labor Robert Collyer was asked by Senator Nickels whether the Reagan administration would seek to turn black lung back to the states, in conformance with the original concept of the law and as John Erlenborn continued to urge.[61] Collyer said the administration opposed such a move on grounds that the states had had the opportunity to pass acceptable black lung legislation and had not done so. As such, black lung had become a permanent federal program and should be operated as such.

Though the states had lost any enthusiasm for assuming the black lung program, they did not entirely neglect the issue. It goes beyond the scope of this study to describe the various activities by each of the states with regard to their compensation programs for disabled miners or their survivors.[62] Yet some of the state programs had a substantial impact on the federal program, in part because of the offset issue. They also had an impact on rate making procedures for insurance carriers providing coverage to coal mine operators. An example of this can be found in Kentucky's activity.[63] Between January 1, 1973 and June 30, 1976 miners totally disabled with black lung or survivors were eligible for cash benefits of $60 to $87/week. Benefit payments were limited to 425 weeks. A Special Fund paid 75 percent of these benefits; the balance was the responsibility of the mine operator or an insurer. There was no requirement that the claimant also file for federal benefits, which were generally lower than state benefits. The statute of limitation in Kentucky forced some claimants to seek only federal benefits.

From July 1, 1976 until July 14, 1980, state benefits ranged from $87 to $131/week for totaly disability or death due to pneumoconiosis. Benefits became payable for the miner's lifetime and were not limited to a maximum of 425 weeks. Another significant change required the claimant to file for benefits under the federal black lung program and make a good faith effort to obtain such compensation. Such federal benefits would initially be fully or largely offset so that only state benefits were provided. However, given the escalation built into the federal benefits, and the unindexed nature of state payments, federal payments would eventually begin and gradually represent an increasing and significant fraction of the miner's total benefits. During this period, 80 percent of the benefits paid in Kentucky were paid by state funds (40 percent from the Special Fund, 40 percent from a CWP Fund created by amendments in 1976). The remaining 20 percent of the benefits paid under Kentucky law was the responsibility of the coal operator or insurer.

After July 14, 1980, the Special Fund paid 75 percent of the benefits while the employer or insurer paid 25 percent. (The CWP Fund was rolled into the Special Fund.) Benefits paid to disabled miners were $217/week unless federal benefits were being obtained, in which case the benefit was reduced to $163/week. (Note that this effectively represented a state offset against a federal benefit that itself offsets against the state benefit.) According to the estimates of the National Council on Compensation Insurance, the present value of reserves needed in a Kentucky claim resulted in costs split 51 percent to the Special Fund and 49 percent to the responsible operator.[64]

While the Kentucky law requires that beneficiaries under the state law apply for benefits under the federal law, not all persons have done so. Some individuals have benefits solely from the federal program after having been denied at the state level, or because of some barrier to pursuing a state claim such as a statute of limitation. A survey of the leading coal mine insurers in Kentucky revealed that among benefit recipients, about 20 percent receive only state benefits and 10 percent receive only federal benefits.[65] The remaining 70 percent initially receive state benefits and will receive supplemental federal benefits subsequently.

To summarize, some states, including Kentucky, Virginia, West Virginia and Pennsylvania, have made considerable efforts to build black lung into their state workers' compensation programs. They have not supplanted what has become a permanent federal black lung program under Part C, despite the original vision that this would be a temporary federal role. State benefits are interwoven with federal benefits, creating complications for those setting insurance rates for black lung, or those attempting to evaluate the component costs of the black lung program.

NOTES

1. *Legislative History of the Federal Coal Mine Health and Safety Act of 1969,* Part 2, prepared for the Subcommittee on Labor, U.S. Senate, August 1975, p. 1859.

2. Ibid., p. 1861.

3. R.P. Fairman et al., "Respiratory Status of Surface Coal Miners," *Archives of Environmental Health,* 32, 5 (September/October 1977) pp. 211-215.

4. On this, see the testimony of Dr. James Merchant of NIOSH, Hearings before the Subcommittee on Oversight of the Committee on Ways and Means, U.S. House of Representatives, July 27, September 28, 1981, Serial 97-32, Government Printing Office.

5. *Federal Register,* 20 CFR, 1976, Section 715.101(a) (5).

6. Montel v. Weinberger, 546 F 2d 679 (1976).

7. *Federal Register,* 20 CFR, 1978, Section 725.202(a).

8. *Black Lung Program Manual,* U.S. Department of Labor, February 1980, Chap. 2-600, pp. 2-3.

9. *Legislative History,* p. 1279.

10. Freeman v. Califano, 600 F 2d, 1057.

11. Sexton v. Matthews, 538 F 2d, 88 (1976).

12. McKee v. Director, 11 BRBS 720.729 (1980).

13. A description of claims procedures can be found in *Social Security Bulletin,* October 1971, pp. 13-21.

14. See Hearings before the Committee on Education and Labor, 95th Congress, 1st session, U.S. House of Representatives, March 14-17, 21, 1977, p. 254.

15. See "Black Lung Benefits Program," OWCP Task Force report, December 1976.

16. Much of the BRB's role is spelled out in part II of its *Black Lung Desk Book* (Benefits Review Board, U.S. Department of Labor, August 1981, iv-14). Also see "Establishment and Operation of the Board and Rules of Practice and Procedure," *Federal Register,* 20 CFR Part 801 and 802, September 19, 1978.

17. See Assistant Secretary Elisburg's testimony in Hearings before the Subcommittee on Labor Standards on HR 7745, House of Representatives, 96th Congress, 2nd Session, August-September 1980.

18. Hearings before the Committee on Education and Labor, 95th Congress, 1st Session, House of Representatives, March 14-17, 1977.

19. See U.S. Pipe and Foundry Co. v. Webb, 595 F 2d, 264 (1979).

20. Oversight of the Committee on Ways and Means, House of Representatives, July 27, September 28, 1981, Serial 97-32.

21. Ibid., p. 147.

22. See the testimony of Deputy Under Secretary Collyer, Hearing before the Subcommittee on Labor on S. 1922, U.S. Senate, 97th Congress, 1st Session, December 14, 1981.

23. Testimony of John Erlenborn, ibid., p. 40.

24. Dr. Lorin Kerr, in comments to the U.S. Department of Labor on proposed standards.

25. Hearings before the Committee on Education and Labor, 95th Congress, 1st Session, March 14-17, 21, 1977, p. 60.

26. Elisburg testimony on HR 7745, p. 81.

27. *Assessment of Resource Loss from Black Lung Automated Data Systems,* Final Report, U.S. Department of Labor, Office of the Inspector General, Office of Loss Analysis and Prevention, September 1981, pp. 293-296.

28. *Black Lung Program Manual,* U.S. Department of Labor, February 1980, Chap. 2-800, p. 1.

29. Based on Regulations. See *Federal Register,* 20 CFR 725.492 (1978).

30. For example, see Zamski v. Consolidation Coal Co., 2 BLR 1-1005 (1980).

31. See Truitt v. North American Coal Corp., 10 BRBS 159 (1979).

32. *Black Lung Program Manual,* Chap. 2-800, p. 1.

33. Insurance arrangements are described more fully later in this chapter.

34. These arbitrary rules have been described by several authors. See for example Peter S. Barth with H. Allan Hunt, *Workers' Compensation and Work-Related Illnesses and Diseases* (Cambridge: MIT Press, 1980).

35. See *Black Lung Benefits Act.* Annual Report on Administration of the Act, Department of Labor, 1979.

36. See Section 28 of the Act.

37. *Federal Register,* 20 CFR 725.366.

38. The practices described in this paragraph are taken from the *Black Lung Program Manual,* Chap. 2-1404, revised October 1982.

39. Based on personal interviews with DOL staff.

40. *Black Lung Desk Book,* xiii-3.

41. *Black Lung Benefits Act,* Annual Report on Administration of the Act During Calendar Year 1981, U.S. Department of Labor, 1983.

42. Annual Report, 1978, p. 30.

43. Annual Report, 1979, p. 14.

44. Benefits are described in chapter 6.

45. The experience of these six states is cited by Donald DeCarlo, "Circular to the Members of the Board of Governors of the National Workers' Compensation Reinsurance Pool, et al.," May 12, 1980.

46. Richard Palczynski, proceedings of Black Lung Seminar, National Council on Compensation Insurance, May 19, 1980, p. VI-3 (unpublished).

47. Ibid.

48. See Conning and Company, *Impact of Black Lung Benefits Reform Act of 1977,* September 1979 and May 1980.

49. Hearings before the Committee on Education and Labor, U.S. House of Representatives, 95th Congress, 1st Session, March 14-17, 21, 1977.

50. See *Compendium on Workers' Compensation,* prepared by C. Arthur Williams, Jr. and Peter S. Barth, National Commission on State Workmen's Compensation Laws, Washington, D.C., 1973, chap. 3.

51. Hearings before the Subcommittee on Labor on S. 1922.

52. Despite these differences in effective rates, surface mining has accounted only for about 35 percent of the revenues raised by this tax because of its relative size.

53. Section 3(b) (2).

54. *Federal Register,* August 18, 1978, Section 725.608.

55. For example, see Background Material and Data on Major Programs within the Jurisdiction of the Committee on Ways and Means, 97th Congress, 2d Session, February 18, 1982, p. 241.

56. See *New York Times,* December 16, 1981. The source is given as "The Treasury."

57. See chapter 6 below.

58. His testimony is in Hearings before the Subcommittee on Labor Standards on HR 7745.

59. Ibid., p. 58.

60. Statement of the Alliance of American Insurers, Hearings before the Subcommittee on Labor, Committee on Labor and Human Resources, U.S. Senate, 97th Congress, December 14, 1981.

61. Ibid.

62. The interested reader can get some idea of this by examining the individual annual reports on administering the black lung programs prepared by DOL. Each report identifies pertinent changes in state laws for that period.

63. Much of this description is drawn from DeCarlo, "Circular."

64. Ibid. This assumes the miner's benefits begin in July 1980, that he lives 19.5 years, that his surviving spouse lives 7 more years, that the federal benefit escalates at 6 percent annually, and the discount rate used is 3.5 percent.

65. Ibid.

• 6 •
Dimensions of the Program

Benefits

Benefits are conferred under the law in three basic circumstances. First, benefits can be paid where the living miner is determined to be totally disabled due to pneumoconiosis arising out of coal mine employment. Second, there are survivor benefits where the miner was totally disabled due to pneumoconiosis at the time of death. This category of benefits, which was added in 1972, eliminates the need for the survivor to prove that the cause of death was associated with coal mine employment or any particular type of disease. Indeed, the 1977 amendments eliminated the requirement that a survivor file a claim where a miner who had received benefits died. An automatic entitlement is conferred on eligible survivors. The third category of benefit exists where a miner's death has resulted from pneumoconiosis arising out of coal mine employment.

Almost certainly as an oversight, the 1969 law excluded certain possible survivor beneficiaries, the "double orphan" issue, and was the initial source of pressure to amend the 1969 act. Conservatives in Congress later expressed anger that this worthy set of changes in the law was used by the act's liberal supporters as a way to bring up the law again, serving to further broaden it through a wide range of amendments. In any event, living miners or survivors are entitled to benefits, which are increased as the number of dependents

205

rises. Surviving dependents can include not simply spouses and children, but may extend to dependent parents or siblings of the miner. If the surviving widow remarries, she loses her benefits as a survivor. In the regulations regarding benefit eligibility, the Labor Department announced that it would not discriminate because of sex in setting entitlements. However, surviving spouses are expected to be overwhelmingly female for many years. (See the paragraph preceding the regulation spelled out in 20 CFR 725.201, August 18, 1978.)

In addition to cash benefits, eligible living miners are entitled to medical benefits for expenses arising out of their black lung condition. Prior to 1978, eligibility for such benefits was limited to Part C beneficiaries. The amendments of 1977 allowed a Part B miner beneficiary to file a Part C claim with the Department of Labor and, if allowed, to collect medical benefits under the program. The 1977 change required the Secretary of Health, Education and Welfare to notify all past Part B recipients of their opportunity to seek such benefits under the Part C program, and that they had up to six months to file such claims. The Labor Department has essentially accepted all such claims in a *pro forma* manner where a Part B claim already has been accepted.[1]

There is no benefit for burial expenses under the program. Awards under Part B or C are tax free. Benefit levels are changed if any dependent status changes, if the miner's earnings change (see section on offsets) or to reflect cost-of-living changes. Unlike the vast majority of awards under state workers' compensation laws, past award levels are automatically increased in this law, albeit somewhat indirectly, to reflect price inflation.

Benefits under the Part B program are paid to recipients from the first day of the month in which the claim was filed or the claimant becomes eligible for benefits. No benefits are paid for the period prior to the date of filing.

Under Part C, benefits are based on the date the claim was filed or the date of death or total disability due to pneumoconiosis, whichever is earlier. In no case, however, are benefits to be paid under Part C for the period prior to January 1, 1974. Accrued benefits are based on the rates that prevailed at the time that the worker or survivor was covered. If the Labor Department is unable to establish a date at which total disability began, the date the claim was filed is used.

It is possible for a miner to be given a black lung entitlement while still in coal mining employment or comparable work. (The usual case would involve the 411(c) (3) irrebuttable presumption.) Cash benefits, however, are not paid or are temporarily halted so long as the miner continues or returns to such type of work. When the work ceases benefits are reinstated.

In the U.S., though by no means universally, workers' compensation benefit levels are linked to the disabled or deceased worker's level of earnings. To do this in the case of black lung would have been problematic. Some of the potentially eligible claimants had ceased coal mine employment or any employment years earlier. This would have presented a problem as to what would be the appropriate earnings level to which one could link benefits. For this reason, there was little disagreement on the position that a flat benefit payment be made to recipients that was independent of the level of previous earnings. The level of compensation was set in 1969 at 50 percent of the minimum monthly payment which a federal employee of the GS-2, step 1 level, who is totally disabled and entitled to benefits under the Federal Employees Compensation Act, would receive.

There appears to have been little controversy about the appropriate level of benefits to be paid under black lung since it was set into place by the original statute. Of all the different issues raised since the passage of the act in 1969, the level of benefits has been remarkably absent from the field of conflict. Because the basic benefit level is linked to the wage level of a class of federal employees, periodic increases in these wage levels automatically lift both new and existing payments under black lung.

The basic benefit amount paid to an eligible living miner without dependents is the same as the benefit paid to a surviving spouse who has no dependents. Aside from spouses, other dependent family members of the deceased miner also can be eligible for survivor's benefits. Table 6.1 lists the level of benefits paid under the act from 1969 through 1984.

Table 6.1
Basic Black Lung Monthly Benefit Amounts
Parts B and C

| Effective dates | Living miner or widow | Beneficiary combination | |
		+1 dependent	+3 dependents or more
12/69 - 12/70	$144.50	$216.70	$288.90
1/71 - 12/71	153.10	229.60	306.10
1/72 - 9/72	161.50	242.20	322.90
10/72 - 9/73	169.80	254.70	339.50
10/73 - 9/94	177.60	266.40	355.20
10/74 - 9/75	187.40	281.10	374.80
10/75 - 9/76	196.80	295.20	393.50
10/76 - 9/77	205.40	308.10	410.80
10/77 - 9/78	219.90	329.80	439.70
10/78 - 9/79	232.00	348.00	463.90
10/79 - 9/80	254.00	381.00	508.00
10/80 - 9/81	279.80	419.60	559.50
10/81 - 9/82	293.20	439.80	586.40
10/82 - 12/83	304.90	457.40	609.80
1/84 - 12/84	317.10	475.60	634.20

SOURCES: U.S. Department of Labor Program Manual and Annual Reports.

The basic benefit amount, paid to the living miner or surviving spouse without dependents, is increased by 50 percent with one dependent, by 75 percent with two dependents, e.g., a living miner, his wife and one child present, and by 100 percent with three or more dependents.

Table 6.2 shows the actual average monthly sums paid to individual recipients from 1970 to 1984.

Table 6.2
Average Monthly Benefits Paid
Black Lung Program Part B

December	Total	Miners[a]	Widows and other survivors[b]
1970	$181.90	$200.10	$149.80
1971	188.50	212.80	160.60
1972	199.40	225.20	169.60
1973	224.30	252.80	187.70
1974	235.40	266.70	196.00
1975	247.70	281.70	207.30
1976	257.40	294.30	216.40
1977	274.70	316.90	231.20
1978	289.40	337.80	243.40
1979	313.20	368.70	264.20
1980	342.50	406.10	290.40
1981	356.20	425.10	303.70
1982	367.70	441.90	315.20
1983	364.80	441.40	314.60
1984	376.40	458.00	326.70

SOURCE: *Social Security Bulletin,* August 1985, p. 80.

a. Includes benefits for dependent wife and/or child.

b. Includes benefits for dependent child of widow, surviving child, parent, brother and sister.

One way to roughly gauge the generosity of the payments under the black lung program is to compare them to other transfer payment programs of the same time period. Table

6.3 lists average actual monthly payments under the retirement and disability portions of OASDHI and a welfare program. Benefits paid under the black lung program appear to be in line with social security benefits, though growing at a slower rate than OASDHI, and well above benefits paid under the old age assistance welfare program (SSI since 1974). Moreover, the President's Commission on Coal estimated in 1980 that a miner receiving black lung benefits plus a miner's pension and social security retirement benefits could earn up to $1,000 per month, most of it in tax free income.[2]

By an alternative measure, black lung benefits do not look particularly generous. Table 6.4 shows the benefits available under state workers' compensation laws in the seven major beneficiary states for two years of the program compared with black lung benefits. While direct comparisons are difficult, the table indicates that in almost all cases, in all of the seven states, workers would have been better off receiving state legislated benefits, assuming they could have collected them. The state and federal benefits are indicated for claims involving death or permanent and total disability. In most state workers' compensation laws, such cases would involve compensating workers or survivors at two-thirds of the workers' previous wages, subject to a benefit minimum and maximum. Typically, these benefits can be paid for the workers' lifetime or that of the survivor, except where there is remarriage. For purposes of comparison, all benefit levels in table 6.4 are based on the assumption that there are no dependents. Federal black lung benefits are larger than the minimum benefits in three states (Kentucky, Virginia, Alabama) in 1982 and above the minimum in those three and Pennsylvania and West Virginia in 1976. However, the federal benefit is consistently far below the maximum benefit levels in all these states in both years. Where miners were working regularly, their wages would have made most of

Table 6.3
Average Monthly Benefits-Current Payment Status
OASDHI and SSI Programs

Year	Retired-worker families		Disabled worker families		Old age assistance SSI
	(Male) worker only	Worker and wife	(Male) worker only	Worker and spouse	
1970	$128.70	$198.90	$136.30	$199.20	$ 77.65
1971	143.70	222.30	152.69	221.60	77.50
1972	177.00	275.20	188.20	274.20	79.95
1973	180.10	276.70	192.80	278.60	76.15
1974	204.20	312.30	217.80	314.00	92.30
1975	225.50	343.90	240.00	344.00	90.90
1976	245.10	373.10	261.40	377.00	94.37
1977	265.90	404.40	283.80	407.50	96.62
1978	288.90	437.50	308.50	443.00	100.43
1979	324.00	488.60	343.60	497.10	122.67
1980	377.10	566.60	396.20	573.00	128.20
1981	N.A.	N.A.	N.A.	N.A.	137.81
1982	465.60	702.50	474.20	690.70	145.69
1983	490.00	742.90	490.90	716.20	157.80

SOURCE: *Social Security Bulletin*, Annual Statistical Supplement, 1984-85, tables 108 and 167.

them eligible for maximum, or near maximum, benefits under the state workers' compensation programs.

Table 6.4
Minimum and Maximum Weekly Benefits
State Workers' Compensation Programs
Seven Coal Mining States and Federal Black Lung

| | January 1, 1976 | | January 1, 1982 | |
Jurisdiction	Death[a]	Permanent total disability[b]	Death[a]	Permanent total disability[b]
Alabama	$ 38- 77	$ 38-102	$ 60-161	$ 60-161
Illinois	103-305	103-205	151-403	151-403
Kentucky	32- 80	32- 96	51-127	51-254
Ohio	93-186	93-186	149-298	149-248
Pennsylvania	94- 95	62-187	142-284	142-284
Virginia	37-149	37-149	58-231	58-231
West Virginia	45-173	45-173	92-276	92-276
Federal black lung	68- 68	68- 68	45- 45	45- 45

SOURCES: *Analysis of Workers' Compensation Laws,* 1976 and 1982 editions, prepared by U.S. Chamber of Commerce. Federal black lung, see table 6.2

a. Spouse only.

b. No dependents.

Miners or survivors were eligible to collect retroactive benefits in several instances under black lung. Under Part C, if the death or disability preceded the date the claim was filed, the earlier of the two was the entitlement date, but not prior to January 1, 1974. In a case where a claim was initially denied but later was determined to be compensable, a long time gap may have been involved. This was particularly important where the law forced SSA and the Labor Department to re-review claims previously denied. For example, where a miner's claim was made between January 1, 1970 and December 31, 1973, where there were three dependents, and where the claim was accepted as of January 1, 1979, the miner received $24,000 in retroactive benefits along with his first monthly check. In 1979, a year many previously denied claims were re-reviewed and awarded, the average retroactive benefit, including those for new Part C claims, was about $14,000 per claim. During FY 1981, about one-half of all Part C benefits paid were retroactive payments.

Thus far, benefits under the program have been considered in terms of monthly or annual sums. An alternative way to view the value of a successful black lung claim is as the value of the future stream of benefits, appropriately discounted and taking consideration of future benefit level changes. A 1980 actuarial estimate was that a successful claim would be worth $106,000-176,000 using a 3.5 discount rate. Undiscounted, a successful claim would be valued between $150,000-250,000 (a point estimate of $210,000), assuming a 17-year life expectancy and a 7 percent annual escalation factor.[3] An unpublished estimate in 1982, using Virginia as the state of residence, a 6 percent annual escalation factor and a 3.5 percent discount rate estimated the present value of a claim that year as $215,000.[4]

The disbursement of benefits on an interstate basis clearly reflects the uneven distribution of beneficiaries nationally. There are several ways of demonstrating this. Column one of table 6.5 is the portion of total payments made to recipients in different states on a monthly basis, in December 1981 under the Part B program. On this basis, recipients in two states, Pennsylvania and West Virginia, received almost half the payments made and persons from five states received about 70 percent of the funds disbursed. Under the Part C program about 60 percent of past benefits went to recipients from five states.

Table 6.5
Benefit Payments Under Black Lung
Selective States

State	Proportion of total payments 1 (Percent)	2 (Percent)
Pennsylvania	30	24
West Virginia	17	14
Kentucky	11	7
Illinois.	6	5
Ohio	6	9
Virginia.	6	5
Alabama.	4	3
Tennessee	3	2

Column 1. Monthly Benefits Paid, December 1981. *Social Security Bulletin,* Annual Statistical Supplement, 1981, p. 246 (Part B only).

Column 2. Benefits paid July 1, 1973-December 31, 1981, cumulative, except responsible operator payments. Black Lung Benefits Act, Annual Report for 1981, Employment Standards Administration, p. 19 (Part C only).

That benefit payments under the black lung program were so highly concentrated in a few states is not surprising. In 1960, 1965, and 1970, between 88 percent and 95 percent of all bituminous coal employment in the U.S. was in the seven states shown in table 6.5. (See table 6.6.) Although comparable data are not available for West Virginia for 1950 and 1955, it seems likely that these seven states accounted for approximately 90 percent or more of the bituminous coal employment in those years. Within these seven states, the three that are clearly most important are Pennsylvania, West Virginia and Kentucky. Table 6.6 also indicates the earlier importance of Pennsylvania's anthracite mining employment and its phenomenal decline from 1950 to 1970. Recall that the evidence seems clearly to indicate a higher incidence of complicated and simple CWP in anthracite miners than in bituminous miners. For both reasons, Pennsylvania's predominance over West Virginia and Kentucky in terms of beneficiary payments in table 6.5 is reasonable.

Table 6.6
Employment in Bituminous and Lignite Coal Mining
The U.S., Selected States, Selected Years
(In thousands)

State	Years				
	1950	1955	1960	1965	1970
Pennsylvania	85.1 (23)	49.7 (23)	31.2 (18)	24.7 (19)	24.1 (17)
Pennsylvania[a]	75.1	30.9	14.9	9.5	5.5
West Virginia	N.A.	N.A.	51.0 (30)	42.4 (32)	45.3 (32)
Kentucky	51.4 (14)[b]	31.6 (14)	26.5 (16)	23.1 (18)	22.7 (16)
Illinois	28.2 (8)	13.0 (6)	9.7 (6)	8.6 (7)	9.9 (7)
Ohio	18.8 (5)	11.0 (5)	9.3 (5)	7.6 (6)	9.3 (7)
Virginia	18.7 (5)	12.3 (6)	13.8 (8)	11.5 (9)	12.1 (9)
Alabama	16.4 (4)	9.2 (4)	8.1 (5)	5.5 (4)	5.3 (4)
U.S.	368	219	169	132	140

SOURCES: *Employment and Earnings, States and Areas, 1939-74,* U.S. BLS, Bulletin 1370-11, and *Employment and Earnings, U.S., 1909-75,* U.S. BLS, Bulletin 1312-10.

NOTE: Figures in parentheses are employment in bituminous and lignite coal mining in the state as a percentage of U.S. total employment in bituminous and lignite coal mining.

a. Anthracite coal employment.

b. 1951 data.

Offsets

The black lung program is an exceedingly complicated one. There is probably no more challenging portion of it to describe than the treatment of offsets. While there is an easy temptation to neglect this issue entirely, to succumb to it would be a mistake. An examination of how offsets have been treated reveals a great deal about this law, including the evolving legislative sympathy for the act. The treatment of the offset forces the government to evaluate the context of benefits provided, and to confront the fundamental problem of overlapping private and public programs available through different levels of government and other providers, to say nothing of the role of the tax system.

Describing the offset issue in black lung is particularly complicated for several reasons. First, the issue has been treated quite differently under the Part B and Part C programs. Second, each amendment to the 1969 law brought changes to the matter. Third, the extent of the offset, if any, may vary under either Part B or Part C in any single year due to the following variables: the miner's age, the source of the income, the type of dependent involved, the nature of the disability, to name only a few. Yet one thing is at least very clear; the offset has been a very significant issue in every instance when Congress acted in this area.

Part B Benefits

In the original law, Part B benefits paid to miners or dependents were to be reduced for income from workers' compensation programs, unemployment insurance and disability insurance provided under state law (only five states provided for such benefits). Additionally, benefits for black lung were reduced to the extent the beneficiary had income exceeding the "excess earnings" amount under section 203 of the Social Security Act. This provision paralleled the earnings test for elderly workers seeking old age benefits under the Social Security Act.

The controversial element under Part B developed out of section 224 of the Social Security Act, wherein miners eligible for benefits both for black lung *and* for social security disability (SSDI) could have the former used to offset the latter. According to this provision, which preceded the Black Lung Act, persons disabled after June 1, 1965 who are 62 years of age or younger will have any workers' compensation benefits added to SSDI so as to not exceed a maximum level of benefits. For a person receiving both benefits, the maximum was set at 80 percent of average current earnings prior to disability, or 100 percent of the amount of total family benefits under SSDI, whichever is higher. Where the combined payments would exceed this, SSDI benefits are reduced. While representatives of the miners expressed dissatisfaction with all of the various offsets, the sharpest criticisms were reserved for the SSDI offset. Part B benefits were not workers' compensation, they argued, and the 1965 SSDI offset provision was inapplicable. Thus, the offset forced the issue of explicating the precise purposes of and reasons for the Part B program.

In the 1972 amendments, the SSDI offset was removed by adding the explicit language that Part B "shall not be considered a workmen's compensation law or plan for purposes of section 224" of the Social Security Act. The Senate-backed version of the 1972 amendments represented a compromise of sorts, retaining an offset but only where benefits exceeded 100 percent of the worker's previous earnings. The House version, which succeeded in the Conference Committee, simply eliminated the offset by defining the Part B program so as to be exempt from it. This method also allowed Congress to achieve its end without having to amend the Social Security Act itself. Thus, matters could be left with Congressman Perkins rather than going to some other House committee.

Opponents of this change in the law pointed to the seemingly perverse outcome that the change meant for states providing workers' compensation benefits for miners with CWP. Assume that a miner with a wife and dependent child earns $390/month and is entitled to $244/month in SSDI benefits based on his earnings. Assume that miner A comes from a state that enables him to collect $200/month in workers' compensation for his respiratory illness. Since there is an 80 percent maximum based on his previous earnings of $390/month, the miner can expect to receive $312/month. Because state workers' compensation provides $200/month, the miner would receive only $112 from SSDI, the other $132/month offset against state workers' compensation benefits. Since the miner receives $200/month through the state, and the Part B benefits at this time were below this level, and offsettable against them, there are no black lung benefits. Worker B, with a similar family situation and earnings record comes from a state where no workers' compensation benefits are provided. He receives the $244/month for SSDI and $153 for black lung under Part B for a total of $397/month, $85/month more than worker A. Aside from the lack of equal treatment, critics of the law argued that it punished workers from the more progressive states with better workers' compensation laws.

The 1972 amendments provided that workers could be found to be totally disabled under the law while still being employed.[5] As such the earnings of the miner under Part B were considered in setting his benefit level just as if he were seeking retirement benefits under social security. In 1972, this meant that the first $1,680/year in earnings were exempted, subsequent earnings of $2 meant a $1 loss in benefits, but where earnings exceeded $2,880/year, there was a $1 benefit reduction for each added $1 in earnings.

In summary, by 1972 recipients of Part B benefits were subject to offsets for payments from state workers' compensation, unemployment insurance, state disability insurance and "excess earnings." An exception to the latter offset was that dependent widows and children (but not miners, dependent siblings or parents) were not subject to the excess earnings test. This variety of offsets, combined with the inconsistent treatment of benefits under the separate programs created an incentive for beneficiaries under the Part B program to supplement benefits under the Part C program. By applying to DOL under Part C, benefits lost to various offsets applied under Part B were then paid to the beneficiary, bringing many back to the maximum level of benefits, regardless of their other sources of income.

The 1977 amendments further liberalized the handling of the Part B offsets. Spokesmen for the miners objected to the application of the offset for benefits paid under state workers' compensation laws when the disability was not due to a respiratory disease arising out of coal mine employment. Given the dangers of employment in mining, many miners were receiving workers' compensation for bodily injuries at the same time that they were seeking black lung benefits. This argument would appear to be more potent if Part B were expressly a workers' compensation program. The 1977 amendments eliminated the offset in such cases. Part B benefits to miners are reduced where the miner receives benefits under a state program for disability due to pneumoconiosis. However, where death from pneumoconiosis occurs and triggers a state benefit, there is no corresponding offset of benefits for widows or dependent children in the Part B program. (It is offset under Part C.)

When John Erlenborn testified on the administration bill in December 1981 he reported that there were a considerable number of Part B beneficiaries that were drawing multiple benefits from SSA without any offset.[6] At the time, he reported that 91,000 beneficiaries under Part B were also drawing OASDHI benefits. Specifically, 63,000 were receiving retirement or survivor's benefits, and 28,000 others were getting SSDI benefits alongside Part B.

Part C Benefits

Offsets under the DOL program have been simpler and there is less contention about them than about those under

Part B. The only offsets under Part C have been for workers' compensation benefits under state or federal (including Part B) programs and, until 1981, an "excess earnings" test for dependent brothers, sisters or parents of miners. Only workers' compensation for pneumoconiosis from coal mine employment was offset even in the original law. As expressly a workers' compensation program, there has been only limited objection to the SSDI offset against Part C benefits. At the time of the 1972 amendments, when Congress eliminated the SSDI offset under Part B, the matter was debated and left intact. Later, Congressman Perkins introduced legislation to end this offset and to pay retroactive benefits to those who had lost benefits due to the SSDI offset of Part C benefits. The effort was apparently not a serious one. Objections have also been raised by miners' representatives and Black Lung Associations regarding the "double offset," such that a miner receiving state workers' compensation benefits can have this used to reduce *both* Part C benefits and SSDI. In some cases, this could result in lower total payments than if there were no state payments at all.

The 1981 amendments significantly changed the offset under Part C by applying a social security type "excess earnings" test to miners or their dependent survivors. The compromise that was worked out applies the new rule only to those Part C beneficiaries who filed a claim after December 31, 1981. The large majority of current beneficiaries are unaffected by the change. As of January 1, 1982, exempted earnings were $4,400/year for miners under age 65, $6,000 for miners 65-71 years, and no excess earnings test for miners aged 72 and over. By January 1, 1983, the age to which the earnings test applied dropped to 70. A miner's "excess earnings" are charged to the primary benefit and to the benefits of all other augmentees entitled under that account. The offset is $1 lost for every $2 in earnings above the exempted amount. By contrast, surviving dependents' "excess earnings" are charged only against their own benefits and not those of the other dependents (such as dependent children in the household). These changes brought Part C beneficiaries into conformity with Part B beneficiaries in terms of an earnings test. The 1981 amendments left other existing offsets intact.

Questions have been raised on several occasions about the rigor with which SSA or DOL actually monitored the receipt of potentially offsettable benefits from state sources. Earlier we noted Erlenborn's testimony in 1981 before a Senate committee where he reported that neither SSA nor the Labor Department were rigorously seeking to identify recipients of state benefits for purposes of offsetting federal payments.

Pennsylvania had provided benefits to miners with pneumoconiosis prior to the enactment of the 1969 law. Benefits were paid from general revenues of the state, and were, therefore, not considered to be workers' compensation benefits. In July 1970 the state amended its law so as to reduce or end payments for workers receiving federal black lung benefits. At that point the Social Security Administration restored benefits that were subject to offset for Pennsylvania payments. Part C benefits were never reduced for miners receiving Pennsylvania benefits under that state program.

In summary, the complexity of offset provisions applying to black lung is impressive. It serves to illustrate the variety and overlapping nature of many transfer payment programs and the difficulty of integrating these with various sources of earnings. Black lung is only worse than other areas because of the existence and separate evolution of the Parts B and C.

Supplementary Income

Benefits under the black lung program are not very generous, but they should not be viewed as the sole source of support for miners or their survivors. There are a variety of public disability or retirement programs that may supplement these benefits, only some of which involve the offset of benefits from one source or the other. In addition to these, there may be privately provided income, a significant source being the United Mine Workers of America Health and Retirement Funds. These funds are obtained through collective bargaining between the UMWA and signatory employers.

There are two basic retirement-disability pension plans for miners covered under these funds. The first is the so-called 1950 Pension Plan and Trust covering miners entitled to benefits on or before December 6, 1974, or who last worked in classified jobs for signatory employers on or after December 31, 1975 (or became disabled on or after December 6, 1974). The second plan is the 1974 Pension Plan and Trust covering miners who became disabled or retired after the coverage period of the 1950 plan expired.

A discussion of details of the two plans is beyond the scope of this study.[7] There are several notable features, however, of each plan. Under the 1950 plan, eligibility for retirement benefits required that the miner be 55 years of age and have 20 years of credited service (a variable number of which must be with a signatory employer) or 10 years of credited signatory service beginning on or after May 29, 1949, three of those years beginning on or after January 1, 1971. Depending upon the year of retirement, benefits under the 1950 plan were as follows:

Table 6.7
Monthly Pensions for Mine Workers Who Have
20 Years of Credited Service

Period	Mine workers who are receiving black lung benefits	Mine workers who are not receiving black lung benefits
December 1974-January 1975	$150	$150
January 1975-December 1975	200	200
January 1976-December 1976	215	225
January 1977-March 1978	225	250
April 1978-	275	275

SOURCE: *1950 Pension Plan-Summary Plan Description,* 1978 UMWA Health and Retirement Funds, p. 13.

For a number of years, the miner's pension benefit was itself reduced where a black lung benefit was received. Further, the disability pension under the 1950 and 1974 plans specifically excluded benefits for miners disabled by black lung. Disability benefits are limited to miners suffering a disabling injury in a mine accident that is medically sufficient to enable the worker to receive SSDI. Black lung cannot be included in this category.

Under the 1974 plan, normal retirement age is 62 years, but otherwise eligible miners can begin to draw (actuarially based) reduced benefits at age 55. The formula to calculate benefits under this plan is more complicated than the earlier one and involves a calculation based on the miner's age at retirement (if between 55 and 62 years), the number of years in service as well as when those years were, but does not depend upon whether or not black lung benefits are being received. A miner retiring on or after March 27, 1978 at age 62 could, for example, receive $275/month for 20 years service, $420/month for 30 years service or $570/month for 40 years service.

Several things must be kept in mind regarding these pension benefits. First, most retired miners or survivors under the UMWA programs are covered by the earlier plan, but eventually the 1974 plan will be the dominant one. As of March 1980, there were 12,400 pension recipients under the later plan and 72,000 under the 1950 plan, but the number of beneficiaries under the 1974 program were growing while those under the 1950 program was declining steadily. Second, many miners who are not affiliated with the UMWA may be covered under other pension arrangements, involving collectively bargained plans or otherwise. Additionally, many former miners were or are eligible for retirement or disability pensions based on employment outside the coal mining industry. It is likely, however, that some miners employed or retired have no pension benefits assured to them.

The pension and health programs of the miners under the UMWA agreements have been known to be in serious financial condition for some time. A report by the President's Commission on Coal in 1980 estimated the 1950 Pension Plan's unfunded liability as $1.9 billion.

Annual payments of approximately $2,800 per underground miner and $6,500 per surface miner are required under the Bituminous Coal Wage Agreement to meet current payments for pensions and to provide full funding for past service by the end of 1986. The pension of a miner under the 1950 plan is $275 per month. That liability will be a continuing source of concern to the parties. Member companies of the BCOA are concerned about the extent of their individual liability, and the cost of the 1950 plan is a factor in the UMWA's organizing difficulties.[8]

Problems with adequate funding and apprehension about the future viability of the pension and health plans are not new concerns of miners or observers of the coal industry. The black lung program did not serve simply to supplement the earnings of miners with retirement or disability pensions. It allowed private pension benefits to grow less rapidly than they would have in its absence. It also served to assure some miners or survivors that supplements to social security benefits would exist, regardless of the developments in the pension plan. The problems of funding the health care program under the UMWA plan have been enormous. As a consequence of difficulties and abuses heaped on the scheme from several sides, the plan had to be reorganized and benefits curtailed in the mid-1970s.[9]

The President's Commission on Coal estimated that a miner retired under the 1950 or 1974 plans might be receiving in 1979 the following: $275 per month from their UMWA pension (1950 plan) or $480 per month (the average) under the 1974 plan, plus $295 per month for black lung (assumes one dependent) and $272 per month from their social security retirement benefit (assumes no dependents). Thus, it was not uncommon for miners to receive in excess of $1,000 per month in benefits in 1979 (largely tax free) from three separate sources.

Between March and May of 1983, Audits and Surveys, a contractor retained by the Labor Department, conducted telephone and personal interviews of beneficiaries under the black lung program.[10] One of the purposes of the study was to establish the amount and sources of income that were being received by miner and survivor benefit recipients. The survey provides information solely based on survey responses and only for calendar year 1982. Miners represented 47 percent of the sample group, widows were 52 percent, while surviving dependent children were 1 percent of the respondents. There were 1,771 completed interviews, which included 51 partially completed surveys.

In evaluating the income of beneficiaries, it is necessary to keep in mind that this population is certainly not representative of the U.S. population. A number of factors that set this group apart from others in U.S. society affect how one views their earnings. First, most miners and survivors live in rural areas, where living costs differ (and are likely lower) than for many others. Second, this group on average has very low educational attainment levels. Audits and Surveys reported that only 1 miner in 10 had completed high school and about 3 out of 4 miners had not attended high school. Ideally, one would compare incomes of this population to others in comparable circumstances.

Eighty percent of the miners were 65 years of age or older. Amongst this subset of the miner sample, only 2 percent received income solely from black lung benefits and under 1 percent received only black lung benefits and a private pension. Fifty-five percent of those miners aged 65 and older received both black lung and social security retirement benefits, while another 40 percent received black lung, social security and private pension benefits. The private pension payments came from employer or union retirement plans.

While income from black lung, social security and pensions appeared to be very common for miners, there were relatively few other sources of income that were widely received. Only 6 percent reported wage and salary income for the household in the previous year, 9 percent reported income from assets, 3 percent received black lung benefits under state programs, while 2 percent more received other state workers' compensation payments. Veterans benefits were received by 5 percent of the respondents. Only 1 percent of the miner sample had received general assistance, AFDC or ADC payments or supplemental security income. The mean total household income of miners in 1982 was $11,740.

For the sample of widows, 91 percent received social security benefits in addition to their black lung benefits. Twenty percent of the widows reported receiving benefits under a union or employer retirement plan. Approximately 7 percent were in households with incomes from wages and salaries in 1982. The mean income in 1982 of widows in the program was $8,170.

It is no simple matter to gauge the adequacy or generosity of black lung benefits. In 1982 a miner or widow collecting benefits for the entire year, assuming no offsets, would have collected over $3,500, while a dependent present could have raised the benefit to over $5,300 (see table 6.1). Given the beneficiaries' mean incomes, it is clear that black lung benefits represented a sizable portion of their overall income and kept many individuals or families out of the poverty classification. In 1982, the poverty threshold for unrelated individuals aged 65 or over was $4,600; it was $5,800 for a two person household with the head aged 65 or over.[11] In the entire U.S. in 1982, the median and mean incomes of unrelated individuals 65 years and older who were female were $6,128 and $8,604 respectively.[12] The median and mean incomes nationally for a married couple household, with the head of the household 65 years or older, were $15,305 and $20,372 in 1982.[13]

Claims Volume

An examination of the data on black lung claims and their disposition provides some clues as to the program's fortunes. Perhaps the single most significant aspect of the data is the impressive number of claims put forward for benefits. Granted that the concept of coverage was expanded after the original 1969 law, which meant that surface mining would be covered, or that "miners" actually meant more than miners in a conventional sense, black lung was limited to a single occupation and industry and to a single cluster of diseases.

Moreover, no compensation was paid for temporary or partial disability. Despite these limits, the program drew amazing numbers of applicants.

In examining and evaluating the data on black lung claims, more than the usual cautions need be exercised. All the data shown in this section are taken from SSA or Labor Department reports. The Labor Department, particularly, has had a consistently difficult time in bringing its data system into order. Various reports show inconsistent numbers and, even within the same report, errors can be detected.

A second issue concerns possible double counting of claims. While some of this can be avoided, at least one problem remains. Some claimants who were denied benefits at SSA filed claims subsequently at the Labor Department. To treat each as a separate claim overstates the number of claimants, though it does not overrepresent the caseload of the agencies.

Some of the data are defined in ways that are not obvious. For example, for several years the Labor Department distinguished between a claim *filed* and a claim *received.* The distinction reflected the Department's sensitivity to its huge backlogs and the problems it had in *receiving* claims that were filed in SSA local offices. This aside, certain claims received by the Labor Department required virtually no decisionmaking by the Department and ought not be treated as part of its adjudicatory caseload.

Another issue in understanding the data on claims volume and disposition is the meaning of the decisions reached on a year by year basis. Many reported denials eventually became acceptances based on the re-reviewing processes that the 1972 and 1977 amendments forced SSA and the Labor Department to undertake.

The data on SSA's experience with Part B are shown in table 6.8. Possibly the most striking aspect of it is the huge number of claims by miners or their widows under this program. In particular, note that about one-quarter of a million claims were submitted in the first 12 months of the program. This outpouring of claims emerged from an industry that had an average daily employment level in 1970 of under 145,000 coal miners.

Table 6.8
SSA Claims Volume and Determinations

Date	Cumulative claims filed	Cumulative claims allowed	Cumulative claims denied
December 31, 1970	247,000	N.A.	N.A.
April 30, 1971	286,100	120,400 (49%)	125,400 (51%)
December 31, 1971	347,700	159,500 (49%)	163,000 (51%)
December 31, 1972	432,600	213,100 (62%)[a]	N.A.
December 31, 1973	547,200	340,000 (64%)	207,200 (36%)
December 31, 1974	556,200	356,600 (64%)	199,200 (36%)

SOURCE: Annual Reports to Congress on the Administration of Part B of the Federal Coal Mine Health and Safety Act of 1969, SSA.

NOTE: Numbers in parentheses are calculated as a percentage of claims decided.

a. Calculated as a percent of claims filed.

Prior to the 1972 amendments that required a re-review of denied claims along with eased criteria to be used in deciding these, and pending claims, SSA had approved about one-half of all claims filed. The 1972 amendments caused 42,000 claims to be allowed by December 31, 1972 that had previously been denied or were pending. By the end of 1973, about 108,000 claims had been approved that had been or would have been denied, save for the 1972 amendments. By 1973 and 1974, the average approval rate on claims rose to about 62-64 percent of claims decided over the entire period. Of claims filed by widows, about 75 percent were approved, compared to just under 60 percent of living miner claims. The higher rate of approvals in death cases, many of which involved fatalities that occurred many years earlier, is consistent with the stiffer burden of proof applied to living miners, where current medical examinations and X-rays could be used in evaluating the claim. About 65 percent of the claims filed by the end of 1974 were from living miners.

At the end of 1974, SSA only had responsibility for paying the claims it had approved earlier and providing assistance to the Labor Department as an intake source of claims. SSA's involvement was reactivated by the 1977 amendments, which required it to re-review claims it had earlier denied, subject to the claimant's choice. Previously denied claimants were given the opportunity to have either the Labor Department or SSA conduct the review. Further, the law mandated that denials by SSA on re-review would automatically be sent to the Labor Department where the claim was to be judged by that agency. About 80,000 previously denied claims were re-reviewed by SSA by June 30, 1979, resulting in almost 23,000 newly approved claims. The 28 percent acceptance rate for these claims was considerably higher than the rate anticipated at the time of the 1977 amendments, though it fell below the proportions accepted by SSA in the re-reviewing process after the 1972 amendments. This brought the number of approved claims by SSA to roughly 400,000, with over 70 percent of all claims being accepted sooner or later. Approximately 37,000 denied Part B claimants asked to have the Department of Labor review the claim directly, and about 47,000 denied Part B claimants waived their rights.

Table 6.9 summarizes the experience under the Labor Department's program, excluding several categories of claims. Column 1 represents the new Part C claims reviewed during various time periods. Several aspects of it are noteworthy. First, while there was some bunching of claims in the first 18 months of the program, the numbers are considerably smaller than the explosion of cases that greeted SSA in January 1970. Moreover, after its initial bubble, the annual inflow of new claims varied only between about 19,000 and 25,000 during the the next five years, providing a somewhat stable flow of work. There was a major jump in claims in 1980, probably a reflection of the somewhat eased standards of adjudication that began to be applied in 1978 and were ended in 1980. With considerably tougher standards imposed during 1980, the number of claims fell off sharply in 1981. Miners and survivors had been advised to submit claims before the interim criteria were replaced in 1980 by the tougher, permanent criteria.

Column 2 of table 6.9 is the number of decisions (initial determinations) made by the Labor Department during various years of the program. Two entries are shown in column 2 for each year beginning in 1978. The upper number refers to decisions made on claims filed on or after March 1, 1978, the effective date of the 1977 amendments. The lower entry refers to decisions based on claims that were denied or pending as Part C claims prior to March 1, 1978. Most of these were claims that were re-reviewed because of the requirements imposed by the 1977 amendments. Columns 3 and 4 show the rate of acceptance and denial as a proportion of decisions made in that year.

There are several striking features in table 6.9. Note the very large gap between claims received and decisions in the first 18 months of Labor Department involvement. Following this, the gap grows even wider with more claims received than determinations made during 1975 and 1976. A small whittling down of the backlog occurred in 1977 but 1978

Table 6.9
Department of Labor Claims Volume and Determinations

Date	Claims received	Part C decisions	Approvals	Denials
July 1973 to December 1974	54,273	14,508	640 (04%)	13,868 (96%)
CY 1975	25,280	16,142	1,614 (10%)	14,528 (90%)
CY 1976	24,934	22,629	1,547 (07%)	21,082 (93%)
CY 1977	18,762	20,527	1,943 (09%)	18,584 (91%)
CY 1978	20,376	3,999	3,445 (86%)	544 (14%)
		3,455[a]	3,433 (98%)	22 (02%)
CY 1979	19,544	18,513	6,843 (37%)	11,670 (63%)
		48,394[a]	24,944 (52%)	23,450 (48%)
CY 1980	39,270	33,764	9,142 (27%)	24,622 (73%)
		67,771[a]	22,898 (34%)	44,873 (66%)
CY 1981	12,605	31,748	5,148 (16%)	26,600 (84%)
		0[a]	0	0
Cumulative	215,000	210,000	78,000 (37%)	132,000 (63%)
		125,299[a]	56,957 (45%)	68,272 (55%)

SOURCE: Department of Labor Annual Reports, 1974-1982.

a. Claims filed prior to March 1, 1978 that were denied or pending as of that date. CY is calendar year.

witnessed a major addition to the inventory of undecided claims. These backlogs reflected the Department's immense difficulties in administering the claims and created very considerable pressure on the agency to move the cases along. By the end of 1978, the Department had received 143,625 claims but made only 77,805 determinations. In the three years beginning in 1979, the Labor Department succeeded in deciding a huge volume of claims, leaving less than 5,000 claims pending by 1982.

One cannot sum the numbers in column 2 of table 6.9 to reach the cumulative number of Part C decisions made because of double counting. Many of the claims that were denied prior to March 1, 1978 were considered again and decided anew after this date. Claims that were appealed where an initial determination was reversed may show up for that reason in more than one year. For these reasons, one also cannot simply sum columns 3 or 4, which reflect the nature of the determinations made by the Labor Department.

Overall, the Labor Department approved about 37 percent of the 210,000 Part C claims that it decided by the end of 1981. Yet, during the first four-and-one-half years of its program, the approval rate of claims decided was only 7.8 percent (5,744 approved of 73,806 claims decided by December 31, 1977). The Labor Department found itself with a large and growing backlog in 1976 and 1977, a very small proportion of claimants being successful, and itself looking particularly harsh when compared to the experience of claimants under the Part B program, particularly after the 1972 amendments. The watershed for the Department was the 1977 amendments. Of the 85,000 decisions based on new claims since March 1, 1978, about 25 percent were approved or about a three times higher approval rate than before the amendments.

The Labor Department was required to re-review almost 120,000 Part C claims because of the 1977 amendments. Of that group of claims, approximately 43 percent were approved. The data do not allow us to separate the approval rates of the previously denied from the claims pending in the Labor Department's backlog on March 1, 1978. The 43 percent figure, however, is much higher than the 28 percent approval rate that the Department of Labor had projected in April 1978.

In table 6.10, data are presented on the Part B claims re-reviewed after the 1977 amendments by the Labor Department. Of the 73,000 claims involved, about 27 percent were approved, also well above the rate forecast for approvals by the Department of Labor in early 1978. The claims reached the Labor Department in one of two ways. Some of them were denied by SSA after a re-review, and then automatically sent to the Labor Department for its review of the claim. In those cases, the claimant was permitted to add evidence to the original file for the Labor Department's review. SSA's re-review was limited to evaluating the existing file only. A second set of claims was not reviewed by SSA but went directly to the Labor Department at the claimant's request. In either case, these 73,000 claims presented similar degrees of effort for the Labor Department to administer, as did the Part C claims re-reviewed after March 1, 1978. In terms of these decisions, taken together with the Part C claims, the Labor Department approved over 98,000 black lung claims (35 percent) out of 283,000 decisions made by it.

In addition to the claims described here, two other sets of cases are sometimes described as claims. It appears inappropriate, however, to pool them with cases requiring a decision on compensability for black lung by the Labor Department. One of these involved the Part B claims that had been approved by SSA, where the claimant sought medical benefits subsequent to the 1977 amendments. Since those benefits were administered by the Labor Department, an application was made to recover certain medical expenses. The basic question of compensability, however, had already been decided by SSA.

Table 6.10
Part B Denials Reviewed by the Department of Labor

Calendar year	Decisions	Approvals	Denials
1979	22,647	7,944 (35%)	14,703 (65%)
1980	33,068	8,027 (24%)	25,041 (76%)
1981	17,520	3,983 (23%)	13,537 (77%)
Cumulative	73,395	19,992 (27%)	53,403 (73%)

SOURCE: Annual Reports, Department of Labor.

The second set of cases involved claims approved by SSA subsequent to the 1977 amendments. If approved, the claims were put into payment status through the Labor Department, the majority of them involving claims against the Trust Fund. The Labor Department reported these as claims, yet they involved little decisionmaking by the Department.

The number of beneficiaries in the program has risen considerably under Part C as the Department of Labor eventually reduced its large backlog. In calendar year 1981, there were 95,135 primary beneficiaries under the DOL program.[14] Of these, 63,000 were living miners, 31,000 were surviving spouses, and under 2,000 beneficiaries were dependent survivors who were not spouses. SSA's beneficiaries, as of December 31, 1981 numbered 376,500, of which 111,200 were miners, 146,200 were widows and the balance of 119,100 were dependents.

The data in table 6.11 reflect the extent to which (successful) claimants were clustered in a few of the coal mining

Table 6.11
Received (Processed) and Allowed Claims by State

Part B Program as of December 31, 1974	
Processed claims	**Allowed claims**
U.S. total	555,842 (100%)	356,642 (100%)
Pennsylvania	163,740 (29) (29%)[a]	124,014 (35) (35%)[a]
West Virginia	101,583 (18) (47%)	59,903 (17) (52%)
Kentucky	60,294 (11) (58%)	32,847 (09) (61%)
Illinois	38,160 (07) (65%)	24,636 (07) (68%)
Ohio	34,270 (06) (71%)	20,100 (06) (74%)
Alabama	29,396 (05) (76%)	15,905 (04) (78%)
Virginia	29,132 (05) (81%)	16,221 (05) (83%)

Part C Program as of December 31, 1981	
Received claims[b]	**Claims in payment 12/31/81**[c]
U.S. total	425,428 (100%)	97,738 (100%)
Pennsylvania	102,737 (24) (24%)	125,473 (27) (27%)
West Virginia	79,009 (17) (41%)	14,531 (16) (43%)
Kentucky	48,676 (11) (55%)	8,311 (09) (52%)
Ohio	37,004 (09) (64%)	9,652 (10) (62%)
Virginia	24,414 (06) (70%)	5,152 (05) (67%)
Illinois	23,387 (05) (75%)	5,249 (06) (73%)
Alabama	22,075 (05) (80%)	3,463 (04) (77%)

SOURCES: Part B-Fifth Annual Report to Congress on the Administration of Part B . . . , p. 8. Part C-Black Lung Benefits Act: Annual Report on Administration of the Act During Calendar Year 1981, submitted 1982, table 2.

a. Percentage cumulated.

b. Includes Medical Benefits Only Claims and Transferred SSA Cases.

c. Includes Trust Fund and Responsible Operator Cases.

states. In the Part B program, 47 percent of all applicants came from two states (Pennsylvania and West Virginia), two-thirds of all claimants came from 4 states, and 7 states were responsible for more than 80 percent of claimants. The allowed claims were even more concentrated, probably reflecting the higher proportion of successful claimants that came from the anthracite regions in Pennsylvania.[15] The data are not precisely comparable for the Part C program, but the Labor Department's claims were almost as geographically concentrated as those in SSA. As of December 31, 1981, Pennsylvania accounted for about one of every four claims, and 7 states were responsible for four out of every five. At that time, payments being made to successful claimants were largely in four states: Pennsylvania, West Virginia, Kentucky, and Ohio.

Costs

Establishing the costs that have occurred under the black lung program is no simple matter. Because the program has been funded by more than one agency, because of the overlap between private and public sector liabilities, with consideration for interest payments on borrowing to support the Trust Fund to name only three complicating factors, it is not possible to take a single figure (or set of figures) and call this the program's cost.

In examining the program's history, at least two elements of program costs are quite clear. First, projections regarding anticipated costs have typically been quite far from the mark, with the largest degree of error usually occurring as members of Congress who supported the law underestimated what program costs would be. Second, by federal standards at least, the program initially appeared to be a very low cost item in the budget, amounting to well under $100 million in the first year and declining thereafter. The smooth sailing that the law's supporters experienced can partly be attributed to the disinterest that most members of Congress showed toward this apparently low cost item in the budget. So long as the bill appeared to be very cheap, and given the very vigorous support for it from key legislators such as Perkins and Randolph, the law understandably found easy going.

Errors in projecting costs of federal programs must be expected, especially when new territory is covered. The black lung area was particularly problematic. First, no one really knew how large the pool of potential applicants would be. This issue depended upon a whole series of unknowns, i.e., precisely what the disease to be covered was, how widespread the disease was, the extent to which people would know of the availability of benefits and submit claims, and the standards of proof imposed by the administering agency. Aside from these difficult questions, cost projections depended upon future benefit levels, which themselves were a function of future inflation rates (since these would trigger pay increases for federal employees, the benchmark for benefit rates). Inflation rates were poorly forecast during the life of the program. Another variable to be considered in any cost projection was the expected number of years that benefits would be paid a claimant. Clearly, this depended on the projected longevity of a group of persons presumably suffering from totally disabling disease. No good assessment of this existed in 1969. What was known, however, was that the Part C program was to terminate by December 30, 1976.

After the Conference Committee had fashioned its version of Title IV of the 1969 law, a vigorous debate occurred on the floor of the House of Representatives between the few foes of the law (that is, the bill that emerged from the conference) and its advocates.[16] Erlenborn said that the original cost estimates had been stated by the law's advocates to be in the range of $30-40 million a year and had been raised to the

$50-60 million range. Secretary of Interior Walter Hickel had written to Senator Javits estimating the costs to the U.S. Treasury of black lung legislation to be in a range from $155 million to $385 million per year, based on the conference bill. Using existing SSDI disability criteria, Hickel forecast that 54,400 miners would be eligible for benefits, and assuming 1.5 dependents each, at $2,657 each, costing $145 million per year. In addition to this, the cost of the survivor's benefit would be about $10 million per year for a total of $155 million, exclusive of any administrative costs.

Assuming a disability standard that was less strict than the one applied under SSDI, Hickel forecast that there would be 140,200 successful living miner claimants at an annual cost of $374 million, plus the same $10 million per year for survivor beneficiaries, or a total of up to $385 million per year. Congressman Perkins charged that these cost estimates were simply scare tactics by the administration to undermine support for the law. Congressman Burton described the Hickel letter as an "ignoble effort" and the cost estimates as "politically motivated." Congressman Dent was the most colorful in speaking to the issue of costs.[17]

Dent estimated that the cost of black lung for living miners would be $32.3 million per year at a maximum. He based his estimate on a miner population of 110,000 persons, noting that only underground miners were susceptible to the disease. He forecast that 3,300 miners would have the disease. By contrast, Representative Collins of Texas argued: "This program will add billions to the federal budget at the time we are trying to achieve a balanced budget so as to halt the inflation facing the country."[18]

On the Senate side, Harrison Williams estimated that about 50,000 miners would receive compensation due to the law. Senator Javits said his estimates for the law were in the $80-100 million per year range, and certainly no more than

$120 million. Presumably, the costs would fall thereafter as recipients died off.

Eugene Mittelman served as Senator Javits staff aide on the 1969 legislation. He reported that the Conference Committee was aware of estimates in the House of a $40 million per year program and estimates voiced in the Senate of $100-120 million per year.[19] According to him, some far higher estimates were expressed in the Conference Committee, but the issue of costs was largely ignored.

As noted earlier, SSA was sorely criticized by black lung supporters prior to the 1972 amendments on the grounds that it was administering the law too severely. Yet, in the light of some of the cost estimates and projections of usage that were made in 1969, these criticisms reflect some inconsistencies or misjudgments by the critics. That is, despite what program advocates charged was an excessive denial rate by SSA, SSA benefits were $110 million, $379 million and $554 million in the first three years of the program. At the time the 1972 amendments were passed (in May), 365,000 claims had been filed with SSA, of which 171,000 were approved and 20,000 were still pending determination. (Many of those disallowed claims would later be approved under the re-review of SSA or the Department of Labor.)

Prior to the passage of the 1972 amendments, the issue of costs arose again. The major source of increase in federal costs due to the amendments was the extension of Part B beyond the original cutoff date. By adding the provision that X-ray evidence alone could not be used to deny claims, the House Committee assumed that SSA costs would increase by about $10 million per year. Opponents of the proposed bill in the House (HR 9212) argued that the program costs were excessive already and would be up to $375 million annually by the end of that fiscal year. (This was itself a substantial underestimate, as benefits paid in calendar year 1971 had already been at this rate; benefits rose by over 46 percent in calendar year 1972.) Moreover, the lack of reliability of the cost estimates made in 1969 was held up now by critics of the attempt to liberalize the law. In response, Congressman Dent completely disregarded the legislative record of 1969 in several respects. First, he asserted that no one had estimated the costs of black lung legislation in 1969. Moreover, he argued, *if* an estimate of $40 million had been made, it applied only to complicated pneumoconiosis as proposed in the House bill. Further,

> Even during debate on the conference report, proponents of the compromise version refrained from making positive statements about the actual cost of the program. The Chairman of the Committee, Mr. Perkins, stated then: "This legislation transcends petty arguments over costs." At the time, I said: "I do not know what the total costs of this provision will be. . . ." In my only specific reference to cost, I was speaking of complicated pneumoconiosis.[20]

Dent's memory clearly proved selective. His "chinchilla coat" argument was made in defense of the Conference Committee's bill, which had dropped the term "complicated" from the earlier House version. Dent's estimates would prove to be at least as far off the mark in 1972 as they were in 1969. First, Dent predicted that the number of claims filed in the first two years of the program, ". . . far and above might be 90 percent of all claims which will ever be considered. . ."[21] He also predicted that the costs of the program would be $190 million in 1972, $135 million in 1973, $231 million in 1974, and $219 million in 1977. At this point, Congressman Erlenborn pointed out that these were not the projected total costs, but one forecast of the incremental increase in costs if HR 9212 was adopted. In fact, the estimates provided by Social Security of the cost implication of HR

9212 were considerably higher than this. Dent tried to deflect the estimates of SSA by asserting that they had prepared five separate, contradictory estimates on the costs of HR 9212, and he blamed them for his own calculation of $40 million as the cost per year of the 1969 law.[22]

Senator Javits forecast an annual cost to the Treasury of $900 million for extending the federal program for 18 months. In fact, this estimate proved to be fairly near the mark.

Table 6.12 contains the estimated cash benefits provided under the Part B program since its inception. The direct payments under the program have remained remarkably stable from 1973 through 1984 at about $1 billion per year. Since the program was turned over to the Department of Labor, three basic factors have affected SSA's payments. First, some re-reviewed cases were subsequently added to its payment roles. Second, cost of living adjustments annually tended to increase overall program costs. Third, declines in the number of beneficiaries due to deaths about balanced off this increase. Thus, by December 1984, the number of Part B beneficiaries was 36 percent below the peak reached in the program in 1974. (See table 6.13.) Most of the decline occurred among miners, where the number of benefit recipients in 1984 was only one-half the number in 1974. From 1974 to 1984, however, average benefit payments under the social security program rose from $235 per month to $376 per month.[23]

In addition to the benefits paid by SSA, the agency incurred certain administrative costs in operating the program. At its maximum, these costs were approximately $38 million, incurred in 1973.[24]

Payments under the Part C program actually could be paid in several ways. First, payments could be made by employers designated as liable responsible operators. In the absence of responsible operators, liability could be that of the Trust Fund established in 1978. Prior to that time, where no responsible operator was identified, payments were made by the U.S. Treasury for the Department of Labor. Additional expenses for the government were incurred in the payment of medical expenses.

Table 6.12
Social Security Expenditures - Part B Program[a]
(In millions)

Calendar year	Benefits paid	Cumulative benefits paid
1970	$ 110	$ 110
1971	379	489
1972	554	1,043
1973	1,045	2,088
1974	951	3,039
1975	948	3,987
1976	963	4,950
1977	944	5,894
1978	965	6,859
1979	983	7,842
1980	1,032	8,874
1981	1,081	9,955
1982	1,076	11,031
1983	1,063	12,094
1984	1,047	13,141

SOURCE: Supplied by SSA to the author.
a. Includes lump sum payments made during the year.

Several matters complicate this picture, however. The Trust Fund or the Treasury have frequently made payments to beneficiaries where a responsible operator denied any liability. In some instances, these employers later repaid the Treasury or the Trust Fund. Further, when the Trust Fund was created, the Treasury was to be repaid for the expen-

244 Dimensions of the Program

ditures incurred by it, both for benefits paid directly by the government under Part C and for administrative costs in operating the program. Since the Trust Fund has been in operating deficit for its entire existence, however, it has had to borrow from the U.S. Treasury to stay afloat. The Treasury has been debiting the Trust Fund's account for interest on this borrowing, adding both to the appearance of near-insolvency that the Fund has lived under since 1978 and to the costs of the program. However, since the Fund is presumably the responsibility of the coal industry, ultimately, the costs of the program may not be borne directly by the U.S. Treasury.

Table 6.13
Number of Beneficiaries - Part B Program
(In thousands)

In December	Total*	Miners	Widows	Dependents
1970	112.0	43.9	24.9	43.1
1971	231.7	77.2	67.4	87.2
1972	299.0	101.8	88.1	109.1
1973	461.5	159.8	124.2	177.5
1974	487.2	169.1	134.7	183.4
1975	482.3	165.4	139.4	177.5
1976	469.7	158.1	143.5	169.1
1977	457.4	148.7	144.5	164.1
1978	440.0	138.7	145.8	155.5
1979	418.9	129.6	146.5	142.9
1980	399.5	120.2	146.6	132.6
1981	376.5	111.2	146.2	119.1
1982	354.6	102.2	144.9	107.5
1983	333.4	93.7	143.0	96.7
1984	313.8	85.7	141.0	87.2

SOURCE: *Social Security Bulletin,* August 1985, table M-34.

*Figures may not sum due to rounding.

The data in table 6.14 reflect payments made for cash and medical benefits under both the Department of Labor and the SSA programs. They do not include benefits paid by mine operators or their insurers, administrative expenses incurred by either agency, or the rather sizable interest expense incurred by the Trust Fund due to its borrowing from the Treasury. Benefit payments do include both regular monthly payments made during the calendar year, as well as lump sum payments in that year where retroactive benefits were awarded. The next to last column of table 6.14 is only one indicator of the program's size. Since the Trust Fund is financed (in theory, at least) by a tonnage tax on coal operators, payments from it cannot be considered a federal obligation—unlike the Part B benefits.

Table 6.14 reveals the very slow start-up of the Part C program as the huge backlog of claims accumulated in the Department of Labor. As the agency began to see its role differently after the 1977 amendments, payments in 1979 jumped by almost 13 times the levels of 1978. Many of these payouts in 1979 and 1980 involved retroactive awards, one of the primary reasons that benefits payments declined thereafter.

An alternative way to focus on some of the costs of the program can be seen in table 6.15. Columns 1 and 2 are the combined Parts B and C benefit payouts to disabled miners and survivors respectively, from 1970 through 1984, exclusive of both medical benefits and payments by responsible operators and their insurers. Benefits to miners peaked twice, first in 1973 when only the SSA program was making payments, and again in 1979 and 1980 after the blockage in the Department of Labor had ended. By contrast, the death benefit program has tended to grow over time. Column 3 is the ratio of death payments to disability payments; by 1984, the ratio hit a peak at over 86 percent. It appears evident that

Table 6.14
Payments to Miner and Survivors, Black Lung Program[a]
(In millions)

Calendar year	Part C benefits			Part B & C benefits including medical[b]	Cumulative
	Cash benefits	Medical benefits	Cash & medical benefits[b]		
1970	$ 0	$ 0	$ 0	$ 110	$ 110
1971	0	0	0	379	489
1972	0	0	0	554	1,043
1973	0	0	0	1,045	2,088
1974	2	1	4	955	3,043
1975	8	2	10	957	4,000
1976	15	3	18	981	4,981
1977	21	2	24	968	5,949
1978	56	2	58	1,023	6,972
1979	715	14	729	1,712	8,684
1980	679	27	707	1,739	10,423
1981	618	35	653	1,735	12,158
1982	545	46	591	1,667	13,825
1983	507	121	628	1,691	15,516
1984	486	108	594	1,641	17,157

SOURCE: Supplied by SSA to the author. Data are consistent with those published in the Social Security Bulletin for all years until 1982, the latest ones available there.

a. Benefits are exclusive of payments made by responsible operators or their insurers.

b. Figures may not sum due to rounding.

the program will soon be as costly in the survivors' area as in the disability area, at least to those beneficiaries supported by SSA and the Trust Fund.

The last two columns in table 6.15 are the ratios of black lung benefit payments from SSA and the Trust Fund as a fraction of all disability and all survivors' benefits (excluding federal black lung payments) under workers' compensation in the United States. Thus, federal black lung payments to living miners were as high as 28.2 percent of the level of all disability payments under workers' compensation programs, excluding black lung in 1973. That proportion fell to 11.2 percent in 1978 but turned upward in 1979 when the Department of Labor began clearing out its backlog. Since then the ratio has declined again, in part due to the continuing increases in benefits paid out under state workers' compensation programs.

In the last column of table 6.15 is the ratio of survivors' benefits paid under the federal programs, excluding responsible operators, to survivors' benefits paid under all workers' compensation programs (excluding federal black lung) in that year. It is notable that in three of the years in the series (1973, 1974, and 1979) more benefits were paid to survivors under federal black lung programs than in all (other) workers' compensation programs in the nation. Indeed, beginning with 1972, the proportion has never been below 80 percent. At one level it seems incredible that death benefits for one class of workers, and for a single (set of) disease(s) should be anywhere near the level of benefits paid for all death claims under workers' compensation in the entire nation. An important ingredient that must be understood, however, is the cost-of-living adjustment for past awards that is built into the federal program but does not exist in most state programs.

Table 6.15

Black Lung Payments, Part B and C
Disability and Death Cases[a]

Calendar year	Cash benefits (in millions)		Survivors/ disability (3)	Disability/ workers' compensation disability (4)	Survivors/ workers' compensation survivors (5)
	Disability (1)	Survivors (2)			
1970	$ 77	$ 33	42.9%	4.6%	16.6%
1971	232	147	63.3%	12.6%	67.7%
1972	330	224	67.9%	16.4%	93.3%
1973	650	395	60.8%	28.2%	144.6%
1974	604	350	57.9%	22.0%	109.4%
1975	595	360	60.5%	18.3%	98.6%
1976	598	380	63.5%	15.8%	88.4%
1977	575	390	67.8%	12.8%	80.4%
1978	591	430	72.8%	11.2%	80.4%
1979	1,033	665	64.4%	16.7%	109.0%
1980	1,077	635	59.0%	14.9%	94.8%
1981	1,030	670	65.0%	12.6%	91.8%
1982	916	705	77.0%	10.3%	88.7%
1983	870	700	80.5%	8.9%	80.5%
1984	823	710	86.3%	N.A.	N.A.

SOURCES: Adapted from Daniel N. Price, "Workers' Compensation: Coverage, Benefits and Costs, 1982," *Social Security Bulletin*, December 1984, table 1; Price, "Workers' Compensation: 1976-80. Benchmark Revision," *Social Security Bulletin*, July 1984, table 3; and data supplied to the author by SSA.

NOTES: Column 3 is column 2/column 1. Column 4 is column 1/all disability payments made under workers' compensation that year, exclusive of black lung. Column 5 is column 2/all death payments made under workers' compensation that year, exclusive of black lung.

a. Excludes medical benefits and responsible operator and their insurer payments.

As the costs of the black lung program mounted steeply, some concerns began to be expressed about them. Supporters of the program argued that the costs were totally appropriate, as they represented a "catchup" for benefits that ought to have been paid under the state workers' compensation programs. Lorin Kerr argued:

> The current annual expenditure of slightly more than $1 billion is scant recognition of the long years of neglect the miners have endured. These payments to living survivors of decades of uncontrolled dust exposure can never equal workmen's compensation payments which should have been initiated in 1943 when Britain first provided such coverage.[25]

A description of the Trust Fund and its activity is found elsewhere in this study.[26] It is in context here, however, to note that projected cost estimates regarding the Trust Fund have also tended to be underestimated. Because the tax was initially set too low, the rates were raised in the 1981 amendments "temporarily." In fiscal years 1980 and 1981, the Trust Fund ran a deficit of over one-half billion dollars a year. In fiscal year 1981, revenue from the coal tonnage tax was only 87 percent of its size in the previous year, and was only approximately 36 percent of the size of the benefits paid that year, to say nothing of coverage for administrative expenses and interest repayment on the $1.5 billion in advances made by the Treasury to the Fund.[27]

In 1980, at a hearing before his committee on proposed amendments, Congressman Carl Perkins downplayed the Trust Fund's problems:

> (The Trust Fund) will come out of the red within the next year and especially 2 or 3 years from today. . . . I would say, within 5 years, the Trust

Fund could easily be solvent. No one knows for certain, but that could easily be the case with the increased production of coal.[28]

At the time of the 1981 amendments, the Department of Labor forecast the impact of the higher taxes and future payouts. Their projections called for the Trust Fund to require advances from the Treasury in fiscal years 1982, 1983 and 1984 of $235 million, $62 million and $37 million respectively, followed by surpluses that would permit full repayment of the accumulated debt, with interest, by 1993. Needless to say, the projections have been well off the mark. In fiscal year 1982, the Treasury was forced to advance $283 million, and in fiscal year 1983, it advanced $358 million more, raising the Trust Fund's accumulated debt to $2.2 billion. Preliminary data for fiscal year 1984 show even a larger deficit and a larger forecasting error than in 1983.[29] The errors in forecasting occurred as benefit payouts were underestimated and projected revenues were seriously overestimated.[30] For fiscal year 1985, coal excise tax collections are in the neighborhood of $576 million, while the forecast had been for revenues of about $700 million.[31] A larger gap than this will likely occur between projected and actual benefit payments.

Data Gaps

The data in tables 6.12 and 6.14 provide only partial estimates of the costs of the black lung program. Unfortunately, hard data do not exist that would permit one to arrive at more complete estimates. There are several basic gaps in the data that ought to be accounted for. First, there are no available estimates of the extent to which insurers and self-insured employers are paying benefits under the federal program. Incredibly, the Labor Department is unable to provide any data on such payments. There are a few clues, however, regarding these payments. Prior to the 1977 amendments, only an insignificant number of responsible operator claims were in payment status. Recall that less than 5 percent of those mine operators who were designated as responsible operators were actually paying benefits, while the balance were involved in appeals. Then, some of the claims that were being paid were transferred to the Trust Fund in 1978. Recall also that the 10,000 or so claims that were switched over from responsible operators to the Trust Fund as a result of the 1981 amendments were probably more than one-half of all the responsible operator claims in that period, and many of these were appealed. Finally, a "rough estimate" by a high level Department of Labor official is that 4 to 6 percent of all claims in current payment status, subsequent to the 1981 amendments, were being paid by responsible operators.

A second gap exists because it is not possible to calculate the costs of state workers' compensation program benefits for black lung. It is useful to recall, however, some evidence based on the survey of black lung beneficiaries.[32] In 1982, about 2 percent of the federal black lung beneficiaries received some state black lung benefits.[33] About 1.5 percent of total money income came from state benefits, compared to 39.5 percent which came from the federal black lung program. However, there is an unknown number of state black lung beneficiaries who receive no federal benefits due to the size of the state benefit and the federal offset provision.

NOTES

1. Regulations regarding medical benefits are spelled out in the *Federal Register,* 20 CFR 725.701 to 725.711.

2. See *The American Coal Miner: A Report on Community and Living Conditions in the Coalfields,* The President's Commission on Coal, Washington: Government Printing Office, 1980.

3. Estimates prepared by Robert A. Brian, *Update-Impact of Black Lung Benefits Reform Act of 1977,* Conning and Company, May 1980.

4. Estimate provided by a national rate-making company in a personal interview.

5. See chapter 3 above.

6. Hearings before the Subcommittee on Labor, Committee on Labor and Human Resources, U.S. Senate, 97th Congress, December 14, 1981.

7. A "Summary Plan Description" of the 1950 and 1974 plans, including various subsequent amendments are published by the UMWA Health and Retirement Funds.

8. *Staff Findings,* The President's Commission on Coal, Washington: Government Printing Office, 1980, p. 56.

9. A description of the problems and the reaction can be found in ibid., p. 83.

10. *A Sample Survey of All Sources of Both Monetary and Non-Monetary Income of Black Lung Beneficiaries,* Final Technical Report, Employment Standards Administration, U.S. Department of Labor, 1983.

11. *Social Security Bulletin,* Annual Statistical Supplement 1984-85, p. 70. For individuals below the age of 65, the poverty thresholds for unrelated individuals or for two person households were $5,000 and $6,500, respectively.

12. "Money and Income of Households, Families and Persons in the U.S., 1982," *Current Population Reports,* Consumer Income Series, P-60, No. 142, p. 82.

13. Ibid., p. 91.

14. *Black Lung Benefits Act.* Annual Report on Administration of the Act During Calendar Year 1981, submitted by the Department of Labor, 1982.

15. See table 6.4.

16. See *Legislative History of the Federal Coal Mine Health and Safety Act of 1969,* Part 1, prepared for the Subcommittee on Labor, U.S. Senate, August 1975, pp. 1541-88.

17. See his reference to chinchilla coats in chapter 1.

18. *Legislative History,* p. 1224.

19. See Eugene Mittelman in *Coal Workers' Pneumoconiosis—Medical Considerations, Some Social Implications,* Mineral Resources and the Environment, Supplementary Report, National Academy of Sciences, Washington, D.C., 1976, pp. 5-6.

20. *Legislative History,* p. 1775.21.

21. Ibid., p. 1781.

22. Ibid., p. 1909.

23. *Social Security Bulletin,* 48, 8 (August 1985), p. 80.

24. Selected Annual Reports to Congress on the Black Lung Benefits Act, U.S. Department of Labor.

25. Lorin E. Kerr in *Coal Workers' Pneumoconiosis,* p. 111.

26. See chapter 5.

27. See *Background Material and Data on Major Programs Within the Jurisdiction of the Committee on Ways and Means,* 97th Congress, 2nd Session, February 18, 1982, pp. 236-241, and Annual Reports to Congress by the Department of Labor.

28. Hearings before the Subcommittee on Labor Standards, Committee on Education and Labor, on HR 7745, House of Representatives, 96th Congress, 2nd Session, August-September 1980, p. 58.

29. See *U.S. Treasury Bulletin* (Summer 1985), table FFO-2.

30. See *Black Lung Benefits Act.* Annual Report to Congress for Calendar Year 1983, Department of Labor, p. 30.

31. See Budget of the U.S. Government, FY 1986.

32. See Supplementary Income section above.

33. *A Sample Survey,* pp. 37 and 377.

• 7 •

Summary and Findings

The 1981 Amendments

The character of the Black Lung Act was changed considerably by the amendments passed in 1981. While the modifications are less dramatic in their impact than one might suppose, looking only at the law this action by the Congress must be considered a significant turning point. At the very least, the series of steps taken to liberalize the law after 1969 were set back.

To understand these amendments requires a realization that a compromise was developed behind the scenes by the contending parties. For perhaps the first time in the history of the law, the executive branch played a vital role in shaping the legislation and served as a counterforce to the program's supporters in the Congress. The basic parameters of the political struggle involved a new administration on one side, pitted against the still influential supporters of the program on the other side led by Congressman Perkins and Senators Byrd, Randolph and Ford. In 1981, the supporters feared that the newly elected president, Ronald Reagan, would seek to scuttle the entire program. The fear was not wholly unjustified. The new president rode into office on a very high wave of public support that permitted him some other significant legislative accomplishments early in his administration. The Senate was Republican-controlled, and the support of his programs by some southern Democrats in the

House of Representatives provided him with substantial strength, if not control, there. Indeed, Congressman John Erlenborn, Perkins' foe on black lung since the Conference Committee report in 1969, hoped to turn the entire program back to the states.

Aside from the fear of Ronald Reagan, the program's advocates were on the defensive in 1981 for other reasons as well. The GAO report on the Social Security Administration's handling of the Part B program had received considerable publicity and had made the program appear to be little more than the coal miners' pork barrel.[1] The GAO was about to issue its report on the Department of Labor's administration of the Part C program and it promised to be highly critical as well.[2] Further, the program was proving to be far costlier than had been forecast, weakening support for it by those outside of the coal-mining states who had previously seen it as a cheap way to deal with the miners. The growing obligations of the Trust Fund and the Treasury's need to continually shore it up dramatized the unanticipated costliness of the program.

Had the administration tried to push through the abolition of the program, or at least ceased accepting new claims, it might have been rebuffed by one or both Houses of Congress. The issue clearly was not a customary conflict between conservatives and liberals or Republicans versus Democrats. In a power fight, the liberal supporters of the program could have counted on substantial assistance from Senators and Representatives from the coal-mining states and areas, some of whom were supporters of the president on most other issues. It is likely that the new president did not want to take on Perkins, Byrd and Randolph in an all-or-nothing conflict. With both sides uncertain of their strength, and mindful of the other legislative struggles yet to come, compromise on this issue seemed both reasonable and inevitable.

In lining up the compromise, several changes that had occurred since the 1977 amendments loomed very large. First, the 1980 regulations issued by the Department of Labor during the Carter administration meant that the interim criteria were no longer to be used. As a result, the approval rate of claims by the Department was certain to drop substantially from where it had been since 1978. Thus, many of the perceived excesses in the program's administration had ended by 1981. Very high priority was to be given by the administration to transferring about 10,000 special cases to the Trust Fund from what had been the liability of responsible operators. This turned out to be an easy compromise to achieve since the United Mine Workers always preferred to have claimants deal with the Trust Fund rather than with responsible operators who vigorously defended their cases.

From the perspective of the program's advocates, perhaps the major change since 1977 was that so many of the old claims had been filed and approved by 1980 or 1981. In a sense, they had accomplished so much already that so long as recipients would not be forced to cease receiving benefits, they had relatively little to lose. In addition, state programs had become much more generous to miner and survivor claimants, in terms both of the likelihood of receiving workers' compensation and the level of their benefits. Thus, the federal program became somewhat less significant to them.

The 1981 amendments consist of two titles. The first is called the Black Lung Benefits Revenue Act of 1981, and the second is the Black Lung Benefits Amendments of 1981. The law was signed by the president on December 29, 1981 to be effective three days later. Title I deals with the Trust Fund and is added to the Internal Revenue Code. Primarily, it raised the tax on coal produced. Additionally it transferred the over 10,000 cases to become the liability of the Trust Fund and not of the responsible operators or their insurers.

Title II modified five sections of the law affecting a claimant's opportunity to successfully seek benefits. First, for claims filed after January 1, 1982, it eliminated the restrictions on the rereading of X-rays by the government's "B" readers. (Section 202(a).) Next, section 202(b) eliminated three presumptions found in section 411(c) of the law, i.e., the 20-year presumption (411(c) (2)), the 15-year rule (411(c) (4)), and the presumption for survivors of miners who worked 25 years or more in the mines prior to June 30, 1971 (411(c) (5)). The fifth change (section 202(c)) modified section 413(b), dealing with the widow's affidavit where no other medical or other evidence existed. It limited the use of such affidavits to persons not eligible for benefits in the claim, that is, to nonself-interested parties.

The 1981 amendments made three significant changes in benefits under the law. First, they limited death benefits in future cases to those instances where the death was due to black lung disease. Second, they provided that federal benefits be offset where the miner had earnings, according to the social security practice. This provision applies only to claims filed after January 1, 1982 and would bring consistency in the treatment of Part B and future Part C beneficiaries. Finally, the change eliminated the Trust Fund's obligation to pay retroactive lump sum benefits in claims where an initial determination of eligibility had been made, but where the responsible operator had contested the award.

The compromise bill was supported by the National Coal Association, representing surface and underground mine operators in the East and West. It was clear, however, that the bill was far from the "complete reform" that they would have liked, thereby causing a split vote by the Association's Board of Directors.[3] The United Mine Workers testified in support of the bill as well.[4] Opposition to the bill came from the Edison Electric Institute, a trade organization of electric utility companies who found the reforms inadequate and the future costs to mine operators unacceptably large. Totally behind the bill was the insurance industry, eager to get off the hook for many of the over 10,000 cases that had been dealt them by the 1977 amendments.

The bill was pushed through Congress in a way that bruised some congressional egos. The bill required unanimous consent to go directly to the Senate floor from subcommittee, so as to be acted on quickly before the session ended. When the bill was then sent to the House, floor debate was limited to 20 minutes and no further amendments were permitted. The straight up and down vote was to be on the Senate bill. The only House committee that played a role in the amendments was Ways and Means, which dealt only with the tax issues prior to forwarding them to the Senate. Clearly, the parties to the compromise had done their homework and wanted no last minute objections or changes to cause the deal to become unglued.

Strikingly, the strongest objections came, once again, from John Erlenborn. Having been forced to swallow the 1969 Conference Committee bill and the equally repugnant 1972 and 1977 amendments, he believed that the 1981 changes were far from adequate to reform the law.[5] His objections, briefly noted here, were directed at:

— the procedures that prevented both adequate debate and the opportunity to amend, as well as the complete bypassing of the House Education and Labor Committee.

— the tax changes, which were completely inadequate to deal with the Trust Fund's financial needs.

— the dropping of the presumptions not applying to the many thousands of pending cases still to be resolved by the Department of Labor. Indeed the 25-year presumption was to be dropped only for those claims filed six months after the law's effective date.

— the extension of the earnings offset under Part C only to future claimants, leaving intact the existing arrangement for scores of thousands of current beneficiaries.

— the rereading of X-rays not being applied to cases pending at the time in the Department of Labor.

— the amendment's failing to change the definition of "total disability" and "pneumoconiosis."

— the transferring of 10,200 claims to the Trust Fund, which would eliminate most, if not all, defense against them.

— the elimination of the affidavit by the self-interested claimant not going far enough. Finding someone else to swear that the deceased miner had respiratory problems would be a simple matter for most claimants.

— the amendments failure to reverse the rule that a negative X-ray could not, by itself, be the basis for a denial of the claim.

Erlenborn's preferences can also be seen in the bill he introduced in that session, HR 4387. However, there was no way he could stand in the way of the compromise that included the mine operators, the United Mine Workers, the Reagan administration and Representative Perkins.

Just prior to the vote on the 1981 amendments, Perkins rose to explain his view of one of the key changes made by the amendments. In so doing, he sought to establish for the legislative record the way that the death benefit provision was to be administered. It also served to reveal the type of dealing that preceded the compromise:

> With respect to the administration's operation of
> the program, the Education and Labor Committee

of the House will continue to monitor it very closely to determine the effect of the changes we are
making by the passage of the legislation today.[6]

With this warning to the Department of Labor, he
stipulated how the bill was to be administered:

A question has been raised regarding the proper interpretation of the provision in the bill relating to
the availability of survivor's benefits in those cases
where the miner's death is unrelated to
pneumoconiosis. We have been very concerned
about the authority in current law to pay survivor's
benefits in those situations; HR 5159, as amended
by the Senate, reflects that concern by eliminating
prospectively the authority to initiate benefit
payments when that happens. The administration
expressed these same concerns. . . .

I want to emphasize, however, that it is not the purpose of HR 5159 . . . to deny benefits when complications of pneumoconiosis have caused a miner's
death or where pneumoconiosis was a substantially
contributing factor to that death. For example,
pneumoconiosis may have been a substantially contributing cause of death in a case where the principal cause of death was pneumonia.

Of course, survivors would not be eligible for
benefits in those situations where death was caused
by a traumatic injury or an unrelated medical condition.

As a procedural matter, a survivor would initially
file a claim for benefits. I understand that the
Labor Department's claims examiners will be in-
structed to give all such claims the highest priority
in developing the evidence necessary to reach a fair

and prompt decision. Once the Labor Department has received medical evidence establishing that pneumoconiosis was the cause of death or a substantially contributing factor to the death, the survivor will receive benefits unless the weight of the evidence developed by the Labor Department's Deputy Commissioner or by a responsible operator establishes the death was unrelated to pneumoconiosis. In cases involving a responsible operator, the burden would, of course, be on it to present medical evidence to rebut evidence by the survivor which otherwise would appear to establish eligibility for benefits.

It is my expectation that the Department of Labor would administer the new law in accordance with this explanation of the survivorship provisions.[7]

With this, Perkins made it exceedingly plain that the Department of Labor was to interpret the cause of death liberally in future survivors' claims. Moreover, for most purposes, the burden of proof rested on the defense. This, of course, meant that either the Labor Department, acting for the Trust Fund, or the responsible operator stood between the widow and her award.

The GAO Reports

Following the enactment of the 1977 amendments, the General Accounting Office (GAO) undertook a review of the administration of the Black Lung law at the request of John Erlenborn. In mid-1980, the GAO published its findings on the administration of the Social Security Administration's portion of the law.[8] The report was highly unfavorable of both the legislation and the manner in which the law was administered by SSA. Most important, the GAO was able to examine a randomly selected sample of claims files and report how actual cases were being decided by SSA.

The GAO study was limited in several respects. It did not examine rejected claims, for example. As such the report sheds no light on why claims were being rejected by SSA, much less whether there was a significant difference between these cases from those that were being accepted. Since no new claims for benefits were being filed under Part B at this time, the study examined cases being re-reviewed as a consequence of the 1977 amendments. Until May 1979, when the sample of 200 files was drawn, SSA had approved 14,789 re-reviewed claims.

In auditing these 200 successful claims, GAO examined the available X-ray evidence, lung function and blood gas studies as reported in the file, medical statements, death certificates, and autopsy reports. In evaluating the lung function studies, the GAO used the test values that had been established originally by SSA for the program. Where a GAO auditor questioned the adequacy of the medical evidence in the file, a consulting physician examined the file also, using the same criteria that all the auditors had used.

The GAO's findings are shown below:

Table 7.1
Benefits Paid To

	Survivor	Living miner	Total
Disability established by medical evidence	15 (11%)	8 (12%)	23 (12%)
Disability established by means other than medical evidence:			
Affidavits	78 (60%)	—	78 (39%)
Inconclusive medical evidence	1 (1%)	61 (88%)	62 (31%)
25 years or more of coal mine employment	37 (28%)	—	37 (19%)
Total	131	69	200

SOURCE: GAO Report, July 28, 1980, p. 8.

According to the GAO's findings, only 12 percent of the successful claims were based on "adequate" medical evidence. It is critical to recognize that this summary finding was not a reflection of SSA's disregard for the law. Instead, it meant that by the medical standards used by GAO, the large bulk of compensated claims lacked medical evidence proving total disability or death due to pneumoconiosis. For example, SSA established compensability in 39 percent of all successful claims (60 percent of the death claims) by accepting statements from persons with a knowledge of the miner's condition. In 68 of these 78 claims, the statements were signed by the claimant, that is, by the recipient of the benefits to be paid under the program. SSA allowed very general or vague statements about the condition to suffice. Of the 78 claims established by affidavit only, the length of coal mine employment was established by affidavit as well in 43 of these cases.

The two examples cited in the GAO report involving the acceptance of survivors' affidavits are reproduced *in toto* below:

— In April 1966, a retired miner died from a coronary occlusion at the age of 82—38 years after the last reported period of coal mine employment. In June 1973, the miner's widow filed a black lung claim stating that her husband had worked over ten years in coal mines and had shortness of breath. Twelve years of coal mining employment was substantiated by a coworker, but there was no medical evidence of disability. SSA approved the claim in January 1979 based on ten years of coal mine employment and the widow's statement of shortness of breath.

The claim had been previously denied twice on the basis that medical evidence did not establish disability. However, under SSA's revised criteria for the 1977 amendments, disability was presumed by affidavit and the claim approved. The only other evidence in the file was a statement by a physician several years before death that the miner's lungs were clear. The widow was awarded a retroactive payment for black lung benefits of $12,240.40 plus a monthly allowance of $232. The retroactive payment was for benefits from January 1, 1974.

— In June 1973, a 54-year-old former miner applied for black lung benefits. On his application he reported 15 years of coal mine employment and listed his disability as "shortness of breath." SSA substantiated four years of coal mine employment. In July 1973, the claimant's physical examination resulted in an X-ray negative for pneumoconiosis and a lung function study that showed no disability. On August 31, 1973, the claimant died of stomach cancer. SSA denied his living-miner claim on September 11, 1973, because of the negative X-ray and lung function study.

On September 10, 1973, the claimant's widow filed a survivor's claim for benefits giving the miner's disability as "shortness of breath." SSA denied the claim in January 1974 and again in October 1978 because of the negative X-ray and lung function study. Although SSA was able to substantiate only four years of coal mine employment, SSA approved the claim in March 1979 on the basis of statements that the coal miner had at least ten years of coal mine employment and had a chronic lung impairment before he died. The only evidence in the file to establish disability was the deceased claimant's and his widow's statements about "shortness of breath."

On March 5, 1979, the day the survivor's claim was approved, the living-miner claim, which had been denied

in September 1973, was again denied by SSA under the
1977 amended eligibility criteria. The widow received a
retroactive lump-sum payment of $22,007.80 and
monthly benefit payments of $348.[10]

According to GAO, 61 of the 69 living miner claims (88
percent) were based upon evidence that was inconclusive. Of
the 61, 56 files (92 percent) contained X-ray evidence of simple pneumoconiosis as determined by the claimant's doctor.
In 23 cases (38 percent) there were physician's comments
about a respiratory or pulmonary disorder, but no other
medical evidence was presented. SSA found that 37 of the 56
X-rays (or 66 percent) did not show evidence of black lung.
Of these 61 claims, 57 (93 percent) had lung function studies
showing no breathing impairment. GAO reports that most
of these claims were accepted on the basis of ten years or
more of coal mine employment, and a positive chest X-ray
for simple pneumoconiosis.

The two claims summaries prepared by GAO involving
living-miner claims are reported below:

— On September 9, 1971, a 58-year-old miner applied for
    black lung benefits, reporting over 20 years of coal
    mine employment and naming his disability as black
    lung. SSA substantiated 13 years of coal mine employ-
    ment through SSA earning records. On October 6,
    1971, the miner had an X-ray taken, which was read
    positive for simple pneumoconiosis by one radiologist
    and negative by two others. The miner had two more
    X-rays taken on February 15, 1972, and May 30, 1974.
    The radiologist who took the X-rays read both of them
    as negative. The miner also had two lung function
    studies made, neither of which met SSA's revised stan-
    dards for establishing disability. A physical examina-
    tion did not show a chronic respiratory or lung disease.

SSA denied the claim in November 1971, January 1972, and August 1973 because of the negative medical evidence. The claim was also denied by an administrative law judge in December 1974. Nevertheless, after the 1977 amendments, the claim was approved because (1) the miner had more than ten years of coal mine employment, (2) an X-ray showed simple pneumoconiosis, and (3) the miner said that he had black lung. The 1977 law precluded SSA from rereading an X-ray interpreted by a qualified reader as showing the presence of pneumoconiosis. The miner received $22,638.90 in a retroactive lump-sum payment and $348 a month.

— On November 10, 1970, a 48-year-old miner applied for black lung benefits. In his application he alleged 12 years of coal mine employment and described his disability to include, among others, his lungs and emphysema. SSA substantiated 6-1/2 years of coal mine employment through employment records. An X-ray taken in 1971 did not identify pneumoconiosis. An X-ray taken in 1973 indicated possible pneumoconiosis. SSA had the X-rays reread in 1974, and they were identified as negative. Lung function tests taken in July 1972 and March 1973 indicated no disability using the revised standards. A blood gas test taken in March 1973 indicated no disability. Physicians' comments during 1971-76, however, indicated lung impairment.

SSA denied the claim in January 1971 and July 1973 because evidence failed to establish a lung impairment. Although SSA was able to substantiate only 6-1/2 years of coal mine employment, SSA approved the claim in April 1979 because the miner states in his claim that he had been employed in coal mines for at least ten years and had a positive X-ray for simple pneumoconiosis. The claims examiner did not consider the negative lung function tests. The miner received $19,404 in a retroactive lump-sum payment and $348 a month.[11]

The final batch of accepted survivor claims involved the use of the 25-year presumption (section 411(c) (5)). Of the 37 claims accepted in accordance with this presumption (28 percent of all the accepted survivor claims) 29 (or 78 percent) had no evidence either of disability or of the presence of black lung. In seven of the other cases, the claimant's radiologist found positive X-ray evidence of simple pneumoconiosis. One claim involved a physician's statement about the deceased miner's pulmonary-respiratory disorder. GAO's description of the two cases they summarized is below:

— On February 10, 1953, a 50-year-old miner was killed from falling slate while working in a coal mine. On February 8, 1971, the miner's widow filed a black lung claim—almost 18 years after the miner died—stating that the miner had worked 32 years in coal mines and that she thought he might have had a lung condition. SSA substantiated 33 years of coal mine employment from his employer.

SSA denied the claim on April 3, 1971, because the miner's death was caused by a broken neck resulting from a mine accident and because the hospital medical examination failed to reveal the presence of black lung or a respirable disease. On April 9, 1973, SSA again denied the claim for the same reasons. The denial was contested by the widow, and on April 10, 1974, the claim was again denied by an administrative law judge.

SSA approved the claim on September 8, 1978, because of the more than 25 years of coal mine employment and no rebutting evidence—death presumed due to black lung. The widow was awarded an $11,776.40 retroactive lump-sum payment and $232 in monthly payments.

— On April 28, 1962, a 55-year-old miner was killed in a coal mining accident. On April 9, 1973, the miner's widow filed a black lung claim stating that the miner had worked 31 years in coal mine employment and that he had shortness of breath. SSA substantiated 29 years of coal mine employment from his employers. SSA denied the claim on June 21, 1973, because (1) the miner was killed in a mine accident, (2) no autopsy was performed, and (3) there was no medical evidence of complicated pneumoconiosis. After the 1977 amendments, SSA approved the claim on August 21, 1978, because over 25 years of coal mine employment established disability for the miner and there was no rebutting evidence. The widow was awarded an $11,092.50 retroactive lump-sum payment and $219.90 in monthly payments.[12]

In evaluating the GAO report, SSA accepted the factual findings of the report and the conclusion in the report, which included: "We believe there was little medical evidence that most of the miners involved in successful awards were totally disabled by or died from black lung."[13] SSA did contend, however, that the legislation allowed claims to be approved without medical evidence of disability or the presence of disease.

Reaction to the GAO report was predictable along the lines of program supporters and critics. Congressman Perkins submitted his views on it for the record.[14] He expressed satisfaction that claims approvals were found to be consistent with the law, but regretted that GAO had substituted its judgment on what ought to be compensated for that of Congress. He criticized GAO for using a purely medical notion of disability and for "ignoring the uniqueness of the coal industry." He also questioned the credentials of the GAO's consultant, whose sole certification was in preventive medicine.

The GAO study of the Department of Labor's program closely matched the one prepared on Part B re-reviewed claims.[15] In a few respects, however, it differed. First, a sample of 50 cases was drawn from each of the nine regional offices that processed DOL claims during the period January-December 1980. Of these, 205 were approved claims. Some of these represented newly filed claims while others were re-reviewed under the 1977 amendments. About 4 percent of these approved claims were filed after March 30, 1980, the date the interim presumptions were replaced by the permanent, and more rigorous criteria.

Using similar criteria to those applied to the SSA claims audit, GAO's findings are shown in table 7.2 below:

Table 7.2
Analysis of Claims Approved
Calendar Year 1980

	Sample		Estimate	
	Number of claims	Percentage	Number of claims	Percentage
Claims approved with inadequate medical evidence:	172	83.9	49,700	83.3
Presumptions	104	50.8	28,900	48.4
Conflicting medical evidence	55	26.8	17,300	29.0
Affidavits	7	3.4	2,000	3.4
Unsupported medical opinion	6	2.9	1,500	2.5
Claims approved with adequate medical evidence	33	16.1	9,900	16.7
Total approved	205	100.0	59,600	100.0

SOURCE: GAO Report, January 1982, p. 10.

According to GAO, about 84 percent of claims approved (172 out of 205) were not based on adequate medical evidence. Included in these were 104 successful claims based almost entirely on the use of the presumptions. While all the presumptions except 411(c) (3) are rebuttable, GAO found that "Labor rarely attempted to rebut these presumptions, even where there was medical evidence indicating that the miners were not disabled from black lung."[16] GAO also reported that "a Labor official told us that Labor was concerned about getting claims approved and that the guidance for rebutting presumptions did not specifically state what type and how much evidence was needed to deny a claim. In addition, numerous Labor field officials told us that because rebuttable evidence was not specifically defined, they ignored medical evidence that could have been used to rebut the claim."[17]

In 27 percent of the approved claims, GAO found that the file contained conflicting medical evidence, and that the preponderance of evidence or the latest medical evidence did not support the claim. GAO found that claims examiners at the Labor Department did not attempt to resolve conflicting medical evidence, instead, giving the benefit to the claimant.

The 1977 Act prohibited the re-reading of X-rays by certified "B" readers. The Labor Department sent claimant's X-rays to such experts, however, to evaluate the quality of the picture. A positive re-reading of a previously judged negative X-ray, however, would be used to support a claimant's application. GAO was able to see the results of 164 re-readings by "B" readers out of the 205 approved claims and match these with the initial X-ray reading.

Note in table 7.3 that over one-third of the X-rays said by the claimant's doctor to show pneumoconiosis were found to be negative by "B" readers. Strikingly, almost 10 percent of those X-rays initially read as negative were seen as positive by the "B" readers. In these cases, however, the claimant could have the benefit of the "B" reader's decision. Thus, "errors" of both types were present, at least as reflected by disputes of the interpretation of chest X-rays.

Table 7.3
Results of "B" Reader Rereading of 164 X-Rays
for the 205 Approved Claims in Our Review

Initial reading	"B" reader rereading	Total	Percent of total
Positive	Negative	57	34.8
Positive	Positive	45	27.4
Negative	Negative	41	25.0
Negative	Positive	16	9.8
	Invalid	*5*	*3.0*
		164	100.0

SOURCE: GAO Report, January 1982, p. 16.

One of two cases cited in the GAO report is repeated here:

— In June 1978, a 70-year-old former miner with ten years established coal mine employment applied to Labor for black lung benefits. In February 1979, the claimant took a pulmonary function test that indicated he was disabled and a blood gas test that indicated he was not. The X-ray taken during the same month was interpreted as positive for pneumoconiosis and reread by a "B" reader in March 1979 as negative. A physician examined the claimant in February 1979 and diagnosed pulmonary fibrosis and chronic bronchitis due to coal mine employment. Labor denied the claim in June 1979, citing a lack of disability and causality, but approved the claim one month later, stating that disability, disease, and causality had been established.

The miner received a retroactive lump-sum payment of $4,799 and a monthly benefit payment of $348.[18]

According to GAO, 7 of the 205 claims were approved based on survivor's affidavit. The file contained no other medical evidence, or the evidence indicated that the miner had not been totally disabled or died due to pneumoconiosis.

GAO found that 6 claims of the 205 awards were based on a physician's medical opinion, with either no accompanying medical evidence, or medical evidence that contradicted the physician's opinion. From GAO's perspective, this was regarded as inadequate medical evidence.

The GAO tracked the experience of 191 miners whom the Labor Department referred to the University of West Virginia Medical Center for testing in 1977 and 1978.[19] Based on these tests, ten of the miners were found to have met the Department's criteria for being totally disabled. By 1980, GAO learned, SSA had approved three claims from this cohort of 191 and the Labor Department approved 97 claims.

The circumstances involving the latter claims are shown in table 7.4.

Table 7.4
GAO Findings of Labor Department Approvals
Medically Tested Cohort

		Approvals
Claims approved by Labor with inadequate medical evidence:		77 (79%)
Presumptions	70	
Conflicting medical evidence	5	
Unsupported medical opinion	2	
Claims approved by Labor with adequate medical evidence		8 (8%)
Claims approved by Labor (unable to locate cases files—information obtained from payment records)		12 (12%)
Total claims approved by Labor		97 (100%)

SOURCE: GAO Report, January 1982, p. 33.

The GAO summarized two of the claims from this group in their report, one of which follows:

— In November 1974, a 62-year-old miner with 13 years proven coal mine employment applied for black lung benefits. In October 1977, the miner had a physical examination, an X-ray, and a pulmonary function test. These tests indicated that the miner did not have black lung or a disabling lung impairment. The doctor who conducted the physical examination concluded that the claimant suffered from chronic bronchitis. In January 1980, the claimant had the same medical tests performed again. The X-ray indicated that the miner did not have evidence of pneumoconiosis. The pulmonary function test met the eligibility test values for disability. The blood gas test showed that the claimant had normal blood gas levels. Labor approved the claim on March 19, 1980, citing the positive pulmonary function test and a presumption of the presence of black lung due to coal mine employment.[20]

The response by the Labor Department to the GAO was similar to SSA's reaction. The audit did not find that the Labor Department was operating inconsistently with the statute. It was clear in both reports that GAO's unhappiness was with the product of congressional action and not with how the agencies administered the law. In both cases, the agencies used their discretionary authority in a manner that favored claimants, i.e., the law was interpreted liberally with respect to them.

The primary reason claims were paid in the absence of adequate medical evidence was that Congress wrote the law precisely to accomplish this. What GAO did not address was why the near impossibility of obtaining conclusive medical evidence for some persons should mean that they would not receive compensation as would occur in traditional workers' compensation systems. Nor did it deal with the difficulties claimants would face in the absence of presumptions where medical evidence or opinion is ambiguous or inconsistent. What the studies do, however, is shed light on the importance of the various devices that were created so as to raise the likelihood that benefits would be paid to claimants.

Conclusions

In several respects, the black lung law was historic. It represented the first tangible step by the federal government to involve itself in activities which, until then, had been left entirely to the states. When viewed in conjunction with section 27 of the Occupational Health and Safety Act of 1970, which created the National Commission on State Workmen's Compensation Laws, it served as a possible forerunner of much greater federal involvement in workers' compensation matters. To the extent that it was viewed this way, the program's successes and failures must be understood as having an impact far beyond the limited area of coal mining and coal workers' pneumoconiosis. It seems highly likely, in retrospect, that the perception of the program's costs and benefits (broadly construed) may have shaped public policy towards other possible areas of federal involvement in compensation.

It is probably simplistic to argue that a generally well received black lung program would have brought about a major federal intrusion into state compensation programs. Certainly, the many interest groups that wish to retain existing state programs are not without considerable political force. Moreover, the very substantial federal expansion into new areas that characterized conditions in the 1960s and early in the next decade seemed to lose its impetus by the latter part of the 1970s. One may only speculate as to how significant this single program has been in shaping a federal policy on workers' compensation. It is not speculative, however, to note that the single area in compensation receiving the most national attention in recent years, that is, asbestos and other long latency diseases, has had a continuing flow of proposed federal legislation without any serious movement towards congressional passage. These bills have all been marked by certain obvious parallels with the black lung law.

In evaluating any law, there exists the problem of identifying its goals. The black lung legislation is especially difficult to nail down since its supporters appeared to have widely differing agendas for it. Clearly, within the Congress there were vastly different perceptions of it. The record makes clear that people such as Senator Javits wanted the program to be temporary in nature, at least after the backlog of "old" cases was dealt with. The convoluted structure of the law, with its separate Part B and Part C programs existed because of the (misplaced) belief that the states would step in and assert their jurisdiction in this area. In retrospect, this judgment proved to be as unsound as the one forecasting that the states would quickly make the federal role under OSHA *de minimus.*

The near frenzy "to do something for the miners" that followed the Farmington, West Virginia catastrophe resulted in the passage of the 1969 law. Support for something beyond simple health and safety legislation was so widespread that virtually no real opposition was mounted to the original compensation provisions. It was only after the Conference Committee reported out its substantial alterations to both the Senate and House versions that considerable controversy developed. It seems clear that the goals of the program varied from those who would at least tolerate a small (inexpensive) program limited to very serious cases of a highly specific and uncommon illness (disabling, complicated CWP in underground coal miners), to those whose goal was far broader.

The reason some of the conservatives gave for limiting the program was a fear that a large scale program could somehow threaten the survival of state workers' compensation programs. Ironically, the reverse has occurred. The greatly enlarged scope of the black lung program together with many of its perceived difficulties, appears to have strengthened the hand of state program supporters. Criticisms that are voiced regarding existing state laws are no longer treated implicitly as a call for federalization. Thus, by having the program grow in its dimensions beyond all the worst fears of 1969, the security of the state programs has become somewhat more assured.

For the ardent supporters of the program, their goal was not simply to enact legislation that *appeared* to benefit members of the coal mining community. If they aimed no higher than that, they could have left matters alone after 1969, or certainly stopped after the time of the 1972 amendments. Instead, they continued to monitor the program closely, and extended it substantially with the 1977 amendments. Indeed, one of the clearest aspects of the program was that its well-placed supporters in the Congress were intent on having the money actually flow to former miners and their survivors. Where administrators exercised any discretion that restricted this flow, the wrath of these supporters was sure to come down on them.

The United Mine Workers of America were neither the most ardent nor the most effective advocates of the black lung program. Initially, the more radicalized Black Lung Associations took the lead in generating support for a program at the local level. With its own leadership problems preoccupying it, the miners' union was almost dragged along into the process, both in West Virginia and nationally. As the leadership problems in the UMWA were gradually resolved, the union reestablished a spokesman's role for itself, and the Black Lung Associations became less influential.

While UMWA leaders could be counted upon to assist congressional supporters in their various reform efforts, it seems clear that the impetus did not come from the union itself. Instead, it was that core of totally committed members within the Congress that responded to the messages being received from their constituents, if and when the program was failing to deliver on its promises.

If one is to learn from the experience of 1969 forward, there are a number of strengths and shortcomings in the program that must be recognized. The following is a brief listing of some of these fundamental characteristics of the program.

The underlying purpose of the program was never made explicit. This inadequacy was more than simply an academic nicety that Congress failed to produce. It led to a variety of problems that shadowed the program throughout its life. For example, was the program to be thought of as a workers' compensation scheme, a specialized supplementary pension program, a disability program, a depressed areas benefits plan, or some type of indemnity or support scheme as in agriculture or under the Trade Adjustment Act to assist victims of a specific industry's decline?

The results of this vagueness that surrounded the program were significant at several levels. First, it generated substantial amounts of ill will by those people, both in and out of Congress, who were willing to tolerate a modest program. By expanding the program at every opportunity, e.g., in the Conference Committee, and with the later amendments, the aspirations of the program's staunchest supporters materialized in a way never envisioned either by them or their opponents. This led, inevitably, to conflict regarding the program.

Perhaps the most serious consequence of the uncertainties regarding the program's aims was the impact on the administrative agencies. It seems clear that neither SSA nor the

Labor Department fully understood what was expected of them, at least until 1972, and probably not until 1978. By 1973, SSA appeared to realize that it was not operating simply a small variation of its Disability Insurance program. The interim standards so lowered the criteria for receipt of benefits, that its Part B program took on more of the aspects of the administratively straightforward old-age program than its disability program.

It was only in 1977 and thereafter that the Labor Department appeared to understand that its mission was to pay benefits quickly, and not to treat each case as a workers' compensation claim. Once that became clear, and the Department was able to promulgate its own interim standards, it was able to comply with the intent of the program's supporters. The uncertainty of the program's aims also affected the miners and their survivors. The evidence is clear that publicity about the program was enormously effective at getting out the claimants. Credit for this goes to the agencies, particularly SSA, to the union, and especially to the Black Lung Associations in the earliest days of the Part B program. It is also clear, however, that the miners and their families may not have understood precisely what their entitlements were. This appears evident from the apparent disappointment that many seemed to experience when their claims were denied or not promptly paid. The measure of this disillusionment can be seen indirectly by the anger that members of Congress expressed and demonstrated towards the program's administrators, in response to criticisms they heard expressed by their constituents. In retrospect, the expectations that were raised in the mining community, partly as a way to alert people to their rights to file claims and probably, in part, to take credit for the program's existence, may have been unrealistic, at least initially. Thus, the program was attacked by some for being too generous and by many others, whose expectations had been raised, for being too tight-fisted and limited.

It is hard to evaluate the black lung program and not be struck by some of its contradictions. No intellectually satisfactory rationale exists for a federal compensation program that is unique to one occupation and to one source of impairment. The reality of its existence can be traced partly to some vague feelings of guilt felt by the public about economic and safety and health conditions in coal mining. Much more influence must be assigned to the political power concentrated in the hands of key people in Congress from the mining states. Perhaps Congressman Dent from Pennsylvania was right on target when he argued that the program warranted support in Congress, just as some of the specific agricultural support programs that had received his vote in the past. This was legislation designed to aid a specific population because a need was clearly present, and the votes were there. While the other groups of workers, survivors or retirees might also be in need of help due to a lack of, or a shortcoming in, appropriate government programs, the votes for them were not there.

Certainly, other serious gaps and shortcomings existed in state workers' compensation programs in the late 1960s, but no federal program was devised to deal with any of them. Moreover, not a single serious study of workers' compensation and pneumoconiosis had been undertaken by 1969. As a result, while the widely accepted notion that the system was not working may have been true, it was not documented at all. Had Congress been willing to have the matter studied prior to its legislative initiative in 1969, it might have found other areas of occupational disease that were inadequately dealt with by existing compensation practices. Certainly asbestos was already well known to be an occupational health disaster.

The question that remains, then, is why the foray into an essentially virgin territory for a single disease and one set of workers? The answer seems quite clear. A larger program, involving broader coverage of industries or diseases, would have run into serious trouble. First, its potential costs would have meant that serious opposition would have come from the Nixon administration. Perhaps, more important, it would have lost some support from those many members of Congress who cared little about coal mining or black lung, and who saw the program as no more than a miniscule tapping of the federal Treasury. A larger scale program also would have brought down on Congress the wrath of all those who were strongly committed to complete retention of the state workers' compensation systems as they existed. Thus, black lung mattered little to most parties so long as it appeared to be both small (in coverage and in dollars) and unique. And by contrast, it mattered a great deal to its very powerful, well-placed supporters in Congress, such as Messrs. Perkins, Flood, Randolph, Byrd et al.

A continuing source of criticism of the program has been of the legislated presumptions found in the law. Again, as the law is regarded by many as a compensation law, it is inevitably compared to the state laws which generally make much less use of presumptions. In the insurance and employer communities, there appears to be disdain, if not hostility for the presumptions found in this federal law. Indeed, the term, presumptions, as associated with black lung, has almost become synonymous with excessive liberality and irresponsible generosity towards workers. It is also held up as an example of what can be expected if an unsophisticated Congress legislates in this area where it has little or no experience. To make matters worse, the presence of the irrebuttable presumption was certain to offend many attorneys who were unaccustomed to such rules in compensation cases and whose legal training seems to make such barriers offensive to them.

There is no need here to argue the merits or the shortcomings of the particular presumptions found in the law. Several points, however, need to be made in hindsight about these presumptions. First, many states had presumptions, including irrebuttable ones, in their laws regarding occupational diseases in 1969 (some of which are still in existence). Since these are not labelled explicitly as presumptions, some persons may not recognize them as such. Yet various rules that limit the rights of workers or survivors to make successful claims in such cases are nothing other than presumptions, some of them irrebuttable, that impose burdens on claimants. Such "artificial barriers" have been in place for many years and seem no less offensive than the presumptions in black lung. Thus, some of the criticism of the principle of having presumptions in the law may be no more than opposition to the ideological character of the law.

An argument for the presence of presumptions in the law, though not necessarily of the ones actually used, probably can be made on grounds of both fairness and efficiency. In terms of the first, a number of circumstances existed that made it difficult, if not impossible, for claimants to provide proof of the kind normally used in compensation programs. This was especially true in claims involving fatalities that occurred in the early years of the program or before 1969. On efficiency grounds, the presumptions enabled many claimants who otherwise would have been compensated anyway, to be dealt with more speedily.

Undoubtedly, administration was simpler and cheaper because of the presumptions, and they helped achieve the goal of the program's advocates, that is, to get money to the miners and their survivors. In one sense, this is confirmed by the behavior of SSA and the Labor Department after they became aware of the real intent of the law. Where claims did not involve responsible operators, the agencies rarely chose to use their legitimate right to rebut the presumptions invoked by claimants. As such, the presumptions served to allow the agencies to comply with the perceived interest of the program's congressional advocates.

Aside from various ambiguities or uncertainties that made the law difficult to rationalize and to administer, the statute created certain contradictions that could not be easily justified. Two of the most obvious of these arose out of the Part B-Part C approach, though they were not a necessary consequence of the split programs. First, there was the period until 1978 when the standards for determining the presence of compensable black lung disease were substantially different in the two agencies. Second, the excessively convoluted approach to offsets meant that recipients of benefits under Part B and Part C were treated differently.

With the benefit of hindsight, the program must be considered as a burden on the integrity of the Congress. Throughout the life of the program, estimates of prospective usage and costs emerging from that branch were off by a wide mark. Had those errors not taken a consistent pattern, one could dismiss them as the simple product of having to work in the dark, that is, a new type of program with no base of experience from which to extrapolate. However, the errors were quite consistent in the direction of forecasting less usage and lower costs than actually were incurred subsequently. This pattern had all the earmarks of disingenuousness on the part of the program advocates in Congress, as they sought to sell their colleagues on the bill or its amendments.

Praise or criticism for much of the black lung program has been directed here consistently towards Congress. Until 1981, the role of the White House was consistently minimal. Perhaps the program was too small to warrant presidential attention. More likely, White House relations with Congress were focused on other issues that could have been upset by some strong involvement by the chief executive. It is also possible that both Democratic and Republican administrators between 1969 and 1980 saw the program as a cheap bone to throw to organized labor, at a time when little else was being made available. For whatever reason or set of reasons, the impetus for and the shape of the legislation were entirely congressional and bore no real marks of the White House.

How successful was the black lung program? If the goal of the program was to get federal money to the coal miner community, primarily to older workers or the survivors of miners, the program was very largely successful. Given the unrestrictive standards applied by SSA after 1972 and by DOL after 1977, it seems totally unlikely that any significant numbers of worthy applicants for benefits were rejected. What seems more likely is that the hundreds of thousands of successful beneficiaries actually exceeded the wildest possible goals set by the program's supporters in 1969. With a significant share of the cost of the program borne by the U.S. Treasury, and with the Trust Fund partly supported by surface mine operators in the West, this was accomplished without too great an economic impact on the underground mine employers. Such was also a goal of many of the program's advocates, especially the ones from the coal mining states.

By most other standards the program was not successful. Surely it is not considered a model workers' compensation program that the states might wish to emulate. Using any conceivable standard, the program was not administered well. Most significantly perhaps, the program has reduced the probability that the federal government will play a significant role in the near future in workers' compensation for occupational disease. Indeed the fact that efforts to create such a federal presence all failed in the 1970s and early 1980s must be attributable in part to the perception that another black lung program, perhaps on a grander scale, would be an expensive blunder.

NOTES

1. Comptroller General's Report to Congress, "Legislation Allows Black Lung Benefits to be Awarded Without Adequate Evidence of Disability," July 28, 1980.

2. Comptroller General's Report to Congress, "Legislation Allows Authorized Benefits Without Adequate Evidence of Black Lung of Disability," January 19, 1982.

3. See Hearings before the Subcommittee on Labor, Committee on Labor and Human Resources, on S. 1922, U.S. Senate, 97th Congress, December 14, 1981.

4. Ibid.

5. His position on S. 1922 can be found in ibid. and in his comments on the House floor on December 16, 1981, *Congressional Record* H 9794-9797.

6. *Congressional Record* H 9792.

7. Ibid.

8. Comptroller General's Report (1980).

9. Ibid., pp. 10-11.

10. Ibid., pp. 11-13.

11. Ibid.

12. Ibid., pp. 13-14.

13. Ibid., p. 14.

14. See the Hearings before the Subcommittee on Labor Standards, Committee on Education and Labor, on HR 7745, House of Representatives, 96th Congress, 2nd Session, August, September 1980.

15. Comptroller General's Report (1980).

16. Ibid., p. 12.

17. Ibid., p. 13.

18. Comptroller General's Report (1982), pp. 17-18.

19. See ibid., Appendix III.

20. Ibid., p. 34.

Index

290

National Study of Coal Workers'
Pneumoconiosis, 66
The New York Times, 12, 24, 202
NIOSH (National Institute for Occupa-
tional Safety and Health), 61, 63,
66, 67, 72, 76, 90, 105, 180, 199
Nixon Administration, 14, 26, 27, 39,
151, 281

Occupational Health and Safety Act of
1970 (OSHA), 275, 276
Ohio, 236, 237
workers' compensation, 214
Old Republic Insurance Co., 175
OWCP (Office of Workers' Compensation Programs) Task Force Report,
200

Palczynski, Richard, 202
Passes, Harold, 87
Peabody Coal Co. v. Director, 137
Pennsylvania, 236, 237
coal mining, 60, 214
workers' compensation, 8, 21, 199,
210, 211, 213, 214, 221
Perkins, Carl, 18, 25, 26, 28, 39, 44,
69, 82, 87, 102, 119, 120, 121, 147,
148, 150, 162, 168, 183, 217, 238,
239, 241, 249, 255, 256, 257, 260,
269, 281
Pneumoconiosis, 55-70
in anthracite coal workers, 56, 60,
214
anthracosis, 55
autopsy, 73, 76, 82, 110, 118, 136,
137
biopsy, 76
blood gas testing, 83, 130, 263,
267, 272, 274
bronchitis, 65
cigarette smoking, 59, 66, 68, 143
complicated CWP, 19, 20, 21, 25,
37, 58, 59, 60, 61, 62, 74, 75, 77,
95

CWP classifications, 57, 62, 63, 71,
72
death certificates, 110, 136
diagnosis, 70-92
evidence, 126, 128-137, 230, 263,
265, 270, 271, 273, 274
miner's asthma, 55
progressive massive fibrosis, 58
silicosis, 55, 57, 58, 65, 67
simple CWP, 57, 59, 61, 62, 73, 74,
75, 266
ventilatory function tests, 85, 86,
87, 117, 129, 130, 263, 267, 274
X-ray evidence, 67, 68, 70, 71, 72,
74, 75, 78, 81, 83, 85, 104, 117,
118, 123, 130, 131, 132, 133,
143, 230, 240, 258, 260, 263,
265, 267, 271, 272, 274
Popick, Bernard, 85, 87
Pneumonia, 261
PL 552 (1952), 7
PL 89-376 (1966), 8
President's Commission on Coal, 30,
104, 210, 224, 225, 252
Presumptions, 80, 85, 86, 97, 98, 101,
109-128, 131, 134, 137, 143, 169,
257, 258, 267, 268, 270, 271, 281,
282
affidavits, 116, 135, 136, 258, 260,
263, 264, 270
interim (see Interim Presumptions)
irrebuttable, 34, 37, 97, 98, 114,
115, 118, 119, 126, 281

Railsback, Thomas, 142
Randolph, Jennings, 14, 28, 39, 40, 83,
238, 255, 256, 281
Rasmussen, Donald, 9, 81
Readers, "A", "B", 72, 74, 75, 130,
131, 132, 258, 267, 271, 272
Reagan, Ronald, 256
Reagan Administration, 159, 197, 260
Renzetti, Attilio, 104